WELLBEING
HAPPINESS
ARCHITECTURE
DESIGN

FRVEN LIM

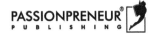

PASSIONPRENEUR®
P U B L I S H I N G

WELLBEING + HAPPINESS THRU' ARCHITECTURE + DESIGN

Crafting Joy and Warmheartedness Thru' Designed Spaces

FRVEN LIM

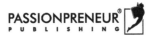

PASSIONPRENEUR® PUBLISHING

Wellbeing + Happiness Thru' Architecture + Design
Copyright © 2023 Frven Lim
First published in 2023

Print: 978-1-76124-130-7
E-book: 978-1-76124-132-1
Hardback: 978-1-76124-131-4

Publishing information
Publishing and design facilitated by Passionpreneur Publishing
A division of Passionpreneur Organization Pty Ltd
ABN: 48640637529

Melbourne, VIC | Australia
www.PassionpreneurPublishing.com

A Dedication to My Teachers

Anyone who can piece together concepts and constructs, including in architecture, has learnt and absorbed knowledge from many others before him. I did not create the knowledge in this book: I fused and married insights and wisdom I was able to glean from experts in different fields. Taking the construction analogy further, my role was to build the bridge that connects architecture+design and the fields of psychology, neuroscience, philosophy and anthropology.

Ideas and lessons simmered for over 10 years before they crystallised into what I now share in this book. I would like to acknowledge the following teachers whose work needs to be credited:

Vishen LAKHIANI: for setting up Mindvalley and sparking the beginning of my personal battle against depression.

Jim KWIK: for your lessons online, which completely transformed my way of reading and my (now) unquenchable thirst for information about the brain.

*Sri Kumar RAO: for the concept of
"no such thing as ultimate reality."*

*Shawn ACHOR: for your revolutionary work
"The Happiness Advantage."*

*(The late) Marian DIAMOND: for your top
brain literally, which helped me to learn
about neuroplasticity in the most stimulating way.*

*His Holiness, the 14th Dalai Lama: for your wisdom and
inspiring me with the concept of "warm-heartedness."*

*Fr Laurence FREEMAN: for your amazing work teaching
meditation and leading the organisation of WCCM.*

*Angelene CHAN: for being my role model for
commitment towards goals, and for guiding me constantly
in the practice of meditation.*

*Mark CANTLE and John O'BRIEN: for the crazy,
seemingly most off-tangent discussions along
the lines of truth and "unfuckwithablity."*

*Ciro NAJLE and Sandra MORRIS: for being my tutors
during the most intensive growth spurt of my
architectural thinking period in 2000, and for teaching me
about the limitless gradations that exist between
the black and white ends of the spectrum for all things.*

AND My Most Personal and Deepest Gratitude to:

GOD: for the twists and turns of my life and guiding me in ways I cannot fathom.

My daughters Ella and Iris: for teaching me what true love and warm-heartedness feels like.

My mother Quek Ing: for the quiet teaching of love beyond all forms of measurable ways.

My sisters, Melinde, Cindy and Elison: for being there for me, especially during my darkest times when what I chose to do was not what you agree with, but you supported me nevertheless.

Claire: for being the mother of my two daughters.

TABLE OF CONTENTS

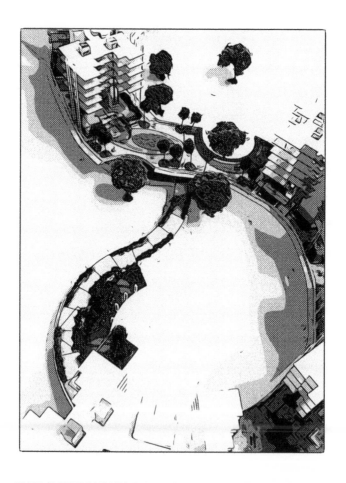

PHOTO (OF STUDY MODEL): CURVES AND NATURED-INSPIRED GEOMETRIES
AS THE ORGANIZING CONCEPT FOR A MEANDERING ELEVATED GARDEN
AT SKY RESIDENCES, WHICH COMPRISES OF OVER 1,300 HOMES.
(LOCATION: DAWSON, SINGAPORE)

Source: Author's own collection

NOTE FROM THE AUTHOR

HOW TO USE THIS
NOT-SO-TYPICAL BOOK

This book is a signature of my rebellious nature. It stamps my declaration of being a disruptor as well as a constructor. I aim to disrupt the long-standing approach to Architecture and Design, which focuses either on functional performance, or on the idolisation of aesthetics and/or imagery. Instead, I aim to construct a conduit that will be the superhighway between experts who know so much about the mind and those who conceptualise the spaces where we dwell every day.

This book is intended to nudge you to look at your life and to understand how it is shaped by the physical environment. It empowers you to make changes, small tweaks here and there, that could transform your life. Because attaining a higher state of well-being, both physical and mental, is a f**king big deal! Only then can you become perpetually on the journey of becoming happier every day.

To truly benefit from it, you need to play full out. You have to process the words, and also take actions. Whatever amount of time commitment you can invest. For yourself and no one else. At the end of each chapter, there are suggestions and also a page to pen your personal insights. Make good use of it.

The end goal: to become happier every day. More joyful than in the 24hrs before. Because this will truly bring you other layers of success, however you define it for yourself.

READING AND LEARNING METHODOLOGY

I encourage the reader to progress through the book from beginning to end. However, being a rebel, and also understanding that this might not be the most convenient or preferred journey, the chapters are also organised to work for anyone who wishes to jump back and forth or only delve into portions which relate to you on any particular day.

If at all possible, I would also recommend you revisit chapters after you have reflected upon their contents. Your mental processing, circumscribing the topic(s) relating to your own personal experience, combined with a re-read, will reveal to you newer insights. If this sounds unbelievable, just try it once, and you will relish the magic.

ARCHITECTURAL WORDS

I have deliberately kept technical jargon and fancy architectural words to the bare minimum because this is not a book to celebrate architecture *per se*. Instead, it is a work intended to anchor the field of design as a medium and conduit through which we can make changes that can affect our states of being.

TWO BOOKS IN ONE

We live in challenging times. Although technological advances and today, AI, seem to outperform us at most tasks and reduce the time we need to perform any task, it seems like we could all do with 36-hour days.

Therefore, I have experimented with writing a book for readers without design training and fused it with another for the architects and designers. In this way, I am building a bridge that links architecture and design with the topics of well-being and happiness. This is a book packed with nuggets of knowledge shared from my personal experiences, and my aim was to blend enjoyment with the pursuit of happiness through the facets of E, G and M (hook here for you to find out more in the book).

FINAL SUGGESTION

Read this book with an attitude of being present. Dedicate small chunks of time but give the words and thoughts your full attention. No multi-tasking. Avoid reading, and then realising that you had not read, and so needing to re-read. This robs you of the happiness of reading.

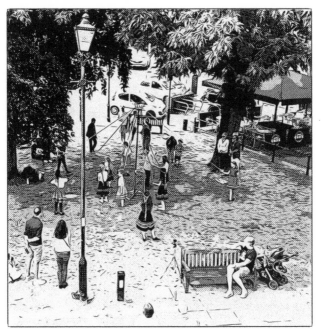

PHOTO: ANNUAL MAYPOLE DANCE AT THE LONDON N21 WINCHMORE
HILL VILLAGE GREEN AT THE BEGINNING OF THE BRITISH SUMMER.

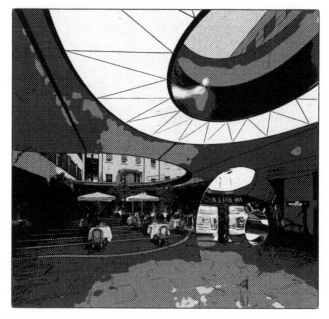

PHOTO: CURVES AND NATURED-INSPIRED GEOMETRIES IN THE DESIGN OF THE COURTYARD SPACE OF THE BILTMORE HOTEL, MAYFAIR, LONDON.

Source: Author's own collection

INTRODUCTION

I am an Architect. In 2010, I was recognised as one of the 20 Architects under the age of 45 who was going to make an impact on the built environment in Singapore and the wider region. Through my professional work, I gathered excellent experience in all scales of urban architecture and spatial design, and hold all the skill sets and credentials to tackle the realm of well-being as a topic.

The technical knowledge is now combined with lessons I have learnt through my own battles with mental challenges. My life's purpose now is to combined these two fields of experiences I have gained, and create the conduit that can serve a much bigger cause: to teach everyone how spaces can impact and help us attain well-being.

RECENT JOURNEY SINCE 2015

In early 2015, my second daughter, Iris, was born, and my family of four relocated back to London from Singapore. That started the second stint of my professional career, and I grew the London office of DP Architects from just one (myself) to a team of almost 12. The growth of the company reflected my ability as an architect and my leadership skills.

THEN THE PANDEMIC STRUCK.

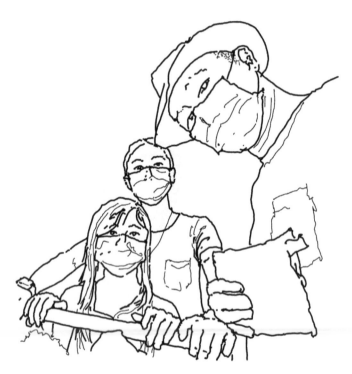

DRAWING: MY TWO DAUGHTERS AND I AT THE AIRPORT
WHEN WE VISITED FAMILY IN SINGAPORE AFTER THE LONG PERIOD
OF LOCK-DOWN AND TRAVEL RESTRICTIONS.

The entire period of my greatest career success started when I was close to 40 years old, with me leading and directing an architectural office of 250 in Singapore. This was in 2011, the same year that Ella, my elder daughter, was born. It lasted until the COVID lockdown at the beginning of 2020. These life events spanned a period of about 10 years and coincided, I realised later, with a long period of chronic depression and self-imposed anxiety.

During this journey, I was constantly investigating how I could contribute to society and trying to balance this with my professional expertise. My focus was to search for ways to figure out how to expand this journey of life, to make it something much bigger and more meaningful.

With the backdrop that I was on the verge of much greater success, becoming a notable person in my industry, the lockdown came and brought me to my worst state. In short, I was suicidal. After having tried all kinds of treatments other than medication, I had no choice but to seek medical assistance. It took about six weeks before I felt like a healthier person – the person who I was, feeling capable of accepting situations, and of facing reality. This was in November 2020. I felt I had the capacity, at last, to sit down and spend time with my daughters.

Gradually, a more balanced mental state became the norm for me, and I conceived the idea of "Small but Big." Today, I describe this experience as like waking up from my longest nightmare.

WAKING UP FROM THE DEEPEST AND DARKEST NIGHTMARE

It felt like I had stood at the edge of a cliff, and taken half a step towards the void. Something pulled me back, and I am now journeying back towards the lush green fields. Two particular heroes helped me start moving on this journey in the dark troubling months at the end of 2020: Vishen Lakhiani and Jim Kwik. Neither of them would know how extensively their online teachings had equipped me to transform my mental makeup, literally dissipating the dark clouds that had previously occupied my skies. The energy I gained through their wisdom and generosity also nudged me towards the state of "unfuckwithability." I have described it - and I really visualise it - as the letting go of layers of worry about how others think of me.

This awakening led me to rediscover that I had the ability to feel joy and to be comfortable that not everything was going to go well. And I was okay with this. Something strange also happened: I started to develop this determination that I was going to use this energy that I had re-composed and channel it, via some method that I had yet to figure out, to spread joy. This was the beginning of the WHAD (Well-being and Happiness through Architecture and Design) movement, which is my effort to increase awareness about how happiness intricately connects with architecture and design. My life journey's twists and turns also led me to think about the possibility that each of us is not meant to just exist, but is meant to serve and support every other member of humanity.

Whatever role or social status we currently hold, I believe we have a strong obligation to contribute towards the betterment of others. We can be a little light that ignites another person's flame and bring warmth to everyone in the room. However, many of us are either not paying attention to this possibility, or are paying too little care to ourselves.

One of the important lessons that I learned through the many episodes of battling with depression and coming out of it, was this: if I allow my own cup to become empty, I would have no love to give to my most loved ones and no chance to serve others. Nothing can be poured from an empty cup. I decided, therefore, that it was just as important, if not more important, for me to always fill my own cup first. We all need to work on this, so that we can then pour forth from our cups.

Why did I write this book?

"I realised that my architectural expertise cannot be limited to the building commissions I take on ... That would be too limited, and fall short of my desire to make a positive dent in the world. The right thing to do is to share my knowledge as widely as I possibly can. Reveal the secrets: What has worked for me can also work for many others."

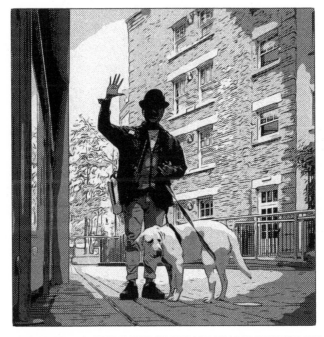

PHOTO: WORKDAY IN CENTRAL LONDON WITH MY LABRADOR RETRIEVER ROXIE.

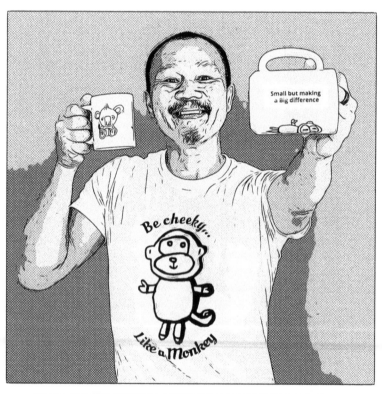

PHOTO: OUR #SBB MERCHANDISE (T-SHIRT AND MUGS) TARGETED FOR ALL
PROFITS TO GO TO UNDERPRIVILEGED CHILDREN CHARITIES.

CHAPTER 1

#SBB:
Small but Big

"DREAM BIG. START SMALL. BUT MOST OF ALL, START."

SIMON SINEK

Many of us may feel we are just one insignificant person in this world of almost eight billion, and that there is no reason why we could have an impact on the community around us. We tell ourselves that it is absurd to dream about changing the world, or making the slightest dent in the universe. We tell ourselves: leave it to the influential and powerful others. I am interested, but I am really not in their league.

In reality, every single small effort starts from the desire to move in that direction in the first place. This book addresses how the seeding of a small intention can lead us to the actualisation of a real movement, regardless of its magnitude.

During the pandemic, all of us were forced into isolation. At the peak of the first lockdown, the rules in the United Kingdom were such that we could only spend time with our immediate family unit. In that period, during the most dramatic roller coaster of my mental well-being, I spent a great deal of time with my two daughters. The three of us together came up with the idea of SBB, which stands for **Small But Big**. The intention here, other than my hidden agenda of trying to increase the ability of my two girls to be empathetic and become aware of how fortunate they are, was to start a small fire. From the smallest sparks.

Without me realising, I was actually starting a new belief and journey, that small things really do have an impact. What is SBB? Basically, it was a project to use the creativity of my two girls to do some good for others. The idea was to create drawings and put them on T-shirts, starting with two iconic hand-drawn pieces by the girls. We wanted to create various types of merchandise and sell it on multiple online platforms, with the intention that all profits would be donated towards underprivileged children.

We eventually donated the profits from the sales of the merchandise to children in Syria through UNICEF. By doing this, my girls understood empathy in action.

As a side note, the important thing to note about social media is that its power is so great that if one is not looking for specific information, one will not find it. The algorithms simply do not provide us with that kind of information. It is unlikely that we will be searching for something like "less privileged." All information on social media is tailored to the user's experience based on their search history. Therefore, children are highly unlikely to be exposed (through social media) to the plight of underprivileged children or people worse off than them. As such, we will naturally not become aware of issues that are not enticing to our materialistic minds, and this can give us a somewhat false impression that such issues are non-existent. This paints an incorrect and misinformed picture of the real world.

I wanted to deal with this and use the **small but big** concept to influence my two girls. The **small but big** idea was born out of my belief that we do not have to be a millionaire to make a difference. We don't have to be a famous person to make a difference, we don't have to have extreme muscular power or to be a super being to make a difference. Much like the butterfly effect,[1] the smallest acts, like the movements of the butterfly's wings, adjusting to the air molecules, can actually have an impact. The theory purports that the butterfly's wing movements can have a domino effect leading to a hurricane or a thunder-storm in another part of the world.

It then dawned on me that positive, well-meaning thoughts themselves do not change anything. Actions do. This said, impulsive actions, or jumping to do the next good deed, would not be sufficient to satisfy my growing appetite to truly make a dent in the universe. We need to bring together psychology, neuro-science, anthropology and various other fields of expertise that relate to our way of living, and the evolution of how this came into the form it is today.

OVERLAPPING DISCIPLINES

For a very long time, the fields of psychol-ogy, neuroscience, anthropology etc. were knowledge sectors residing in their own zones and perhaps discussed amongst scholars. However, I feel strongly that the amalgama-tion of different disciplines can result in some-thing which is a lot more useful. For example, architecture and design layered with psychol-ogy, neuroscience, and general culture can be combined to provide us with new insights, new clues as to how we can uplift our states of well-being using activities and design to influence and shape us. I started thinking about how findings from the research can be applied to improve everyday life.

Small adjustments can make a big impact. The nuances of our belief systems, how we use space and the most subtle tweaks have the power to create brand new habits, and these small new routines can then, in turn, create very big differences in our everyday lives.

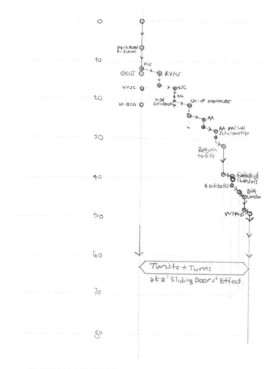

DIAGRAM: MY PERSONAL TRACKING CHART SHOWING REFLECTIONS OF MY LIFE'S TWIST AND TURNS THUS FAR.

MY TWIST AND TURNS

Have you ever thought about how, where, and what you are today might have been different if some things that happened had taken a slightly different course?[2]

Our life experiences affects how we relate to our society and our community. When I was growing up, there were a number of distinct moments when certain decisions and certain events happened that, if they had not occurred, would have changed who I am today.

Here I share my personal journey which even I had forgotten, and only pieced together when writing this book.

MY GRANDFATHER AND I

For about two years or so when I was 10, I would help my grandfather at his makeshift newspaper stall every Saturday and Sunday. I would set out at about 5 pm and walk four bus stops with my grandfather ("Ah Gong") to the local town centre where his stall was located. We would not return until about half an hour before midnight. Those six hours passed rather slowly, sitting with my grandfather at the foot of the overhead bridge diagonally opposite the Bus Interchange. Apparently, this spot was identified to be blessed with a reasonably good footfall of punters who fancied their luck in the local version of "mini-lottery" called 4D (4 digits). From memory, I recall that our commission was 1-2 cents for each newspaper that we sold; a night's work of sit-wait-sell and absolute boredom might bring an income of 2 to 3 Singaporean dollars, equivalent then to the cost of a simple meal of noodles and a drink at the local hawker centres.

In those days, this night venture was something I felt extremely uncomfortable about, to say the least. In my mind, to be selling papers in the evenings indicated that one was poor and of a lower social class. There was always the slight concern that I might bump into people who would recognise me. I reckon my grandfather thought nothing about it at all, given that he had himself been a labourer ("coolie") upon reaching the Singapore shores in his teens. But I did.

Social conditioning had instilled into a young boy's mind that being poor was something to be ashamed of. Until today, I cannot remember much about how I managed to while away all that time, hours twice a week with a man about five decades older who neither spoke much nor expressed any emotions. My grandfather's life had involved a long journey from Fujian, China, running away from being conscripted into the army to fight against the Japanese. It was a one-way trip. He never saw any of his family ever again and, like many others embroiled in the same circumstances, exchanged most of his wages, earned through carrying sacks at the Singapore River go-downs, for opium smoking. It was for him (and countless others) an addiction that lasted till his last breath, but also an escape from the loneliness and emotional burden of missing home. Why am I sharing all these details from my personal journal? I guess I want to disconnect the bullsh*t rule of modern society that financial wealth is the only dedicated aspiration one should strive for.

The more books and research papers I read, the more I feel the urge to dispel longstanding myths. The fact is that happiness and fulfilment come from more complex sources than money. Whilst money does facilitate access to a certain lifestyle, to see it as the ultimate goal is so completely wrong.

Until very recently, I had kept my past very much a secret. I believed that this experience of selling newspapers at a street stall was something to be erased from my memory. It indicated that I belonged to a low-income class, and deserved to be looked down upon in a society that celebrates those who are financially affluent. It is presumed that if you are someone who is notable, or if you are someone who is established, you do not come from a background of selling newspapers with your grandfather.[3]

Of course, I see things completely differently now.

Growing up in Singapore was quite an experience, and it shaped me in many ways. I recall my childhood with a sense of nostalgia, surprised that I was so determined to achieve certain goals.

CHOOSING MY OWN DESTINY

In Singapore, a child typically attends primary school for six years. At the age of 12 I was given the choice of a new school program. The government was trying to challenge the smarter kids. At the time the program was only in its second or third year, and I received an offer for the special assistance programme (SAP): the smartest 10% of Singaporean 12-year-olds would join a secondary school and take up a challenge of being educated in two first languages: English and Chinese, which was the native tongue of my race and ethnicity.

I opted not to choose the SAP because I wanted to start my secondary school education at the Raffles Institution (RI). I had this narrative in my head that anyone who was going to make it in life should come from a well-reputed school such as the RI. It was where all the politicians or anyone who became somebody were educated. My logic was, if I qualify to be in the top 10% of all 12-year-old Singaporean kids, then I should stand a chance of getting into RI.

Guess what? I did qualify, but being right at the cut-off mark, I needed a little luck to get in. As someone who always draws the short straw, I was not selected by the school.

I received a printed note from the Ministry of Education, directing me to another school I was not keen on. If you know anything about the Singapore system, you would understand that one just has to follow and not challenge. And so, on the first day of the new school year, I reported to this assigned school, the one I did not want to go to. Within two or three hours on the first day, I had made up my mind that I was not going to spend my high school years there. I cannot recall vividly what I was thinking, but

I was definitely having some uncomfortable churning in my stomach, perhaps something we call gut instinct, that I was sliding away from my supposed destiny.

I don't know what gave me the courage, but I determinedly proceeded to take a bus and went to one of the special system programme schools, River Valley High School, the one which I would have chosen to go to had I opted for the SAP scheme. All by myself at the age of 12, I arrived at this school and promptly enquired about the location of the Vice Principal's office. I found it, knocked on the door and politely entered. Despite the nervousness, I was outwardly calm and asked to be accepted into that school.

I do not know how, but the response I got from the Vice Principal was a most straight-forward, "Well, you report to this school from tomorrow onwards then." From what I remember, this was for me a most natural and appropriate reply. Why I did not consider it a tad audacious to behave this way, I cannot fathom, even to this day. I recall that incident now, and wonder what led me to be so determined and focused. These sorts of childhood incidents were an indicator of my tendency to achieve whatever I set my mind to. I had the mindset: "If you don't ask, you'll never get it."

I completed my secondary education. And the same thing happened when I was 16: I was unlucky again. Although I could have qualified, I wanted to go to National Junior College, which was where anyone who achieved well in life would have gone for their A-levels education (between the ages of 17 and 18). Again, I was right at the cut-off point for entry, and I was not allocated my choice.

I ended up being assigned to report to another establishment. It just did not feel right, but I thought it would be better if I did not act impulsively. After two hours of validating my predetermined opinion, I decided to take control of my fate again. I journeyed by public transport to National Junior College, not for a minute rethinking my decision. I found the administration office and politely related my circumstances and request to the Vice Principal. A short matter-of-fact meeting later, I received the nod of approval to report to a National Junior College from day two onwards. Hooray! I must have done all of this in one compressed act, holding my breath throughout. Thinking about it today, I am bewildered, and cannot quite explain to myself what came over me to take such a stand.

I was active and I enjoyed those years pursuing my A levels. This was then followed by two and half years of mandatory National military Service.

CREATIVE PURSUITS

During this period, I was fortunate enough to secure a government scholarship to study architecture at the National University of Singapore. I was to start after my army commitments.

But I had always dreamt about being a creative director who would accomplish fame and glory in the advertising industry. This spurred me to invest all the time that I could carve out, during the two and a half years of being in the armed forces, to hunt for some kind of overseas scholarship to give me an opportunity to study in the UK in the field of creative arts. Exposure to Western education was what I wanted. Oddly, "Western" for me meant the United Kingdom. I guess it was the colonial rule of Singapore that influenced me as a 20-year-old. In fact, I was so fascinated by my dream of going overseas, that I did not properly appreciate that I had already received a scholarship in Singapore.

I imagined working into the wee hours, crafting ideas and using visual graphics to communicate concepts and ideas. Like we see in the movies, creative geniuses working all odd hours, having eureka moments. That's what seemed to me to be the perfect career.

Suddenly, it dawned on me that if I was going to study and pursue architecture at the local (Singapore) university, why had I not considered that it was possible to pursue this discipline overseas? It was then that I completely dropped the idea of studying advertising.

It was like a major awakening, and I remember frantically figuring out how this might actually be possible. I realised that the Housing Development Board, which was the Housing Authority of Singapore, could be a patron that I could attempt to secure a scholarship from. I picked up the phone (this was the pre-internet era) and tried to contact someone from the Housing Authority. On the other end of the line was a lady from the human resources department, who then promptly advised me that the scholarship applications had already closed, and that I could put in an application the following year. I explained to her that I was about to complete my National Service.

Something magical happened that moment: she paused, and proceeded to obtain more information about my academic and other qualifications. She said that I technically qualified, and took me off the routine protocol, suggested that I should come in, pick up the forms and fill them in. Upon her advice, various administrative paperwork activities ensued.

Within two weeks, I was invited for an interview, and soon I was informed that they had decided to send me to the UK for an education in architecture. Thinking back, if she had not bothered, I would not have had the chance!

Before leaving Singapore for the UK, I had only been on a single, one-and-a-half-hour flight. Travelling to the UK was a very long trip. A massive deal.

OVERSEAS LEARNINGS

At the University of Manchester architecture school, I was always positioned amongst the top performers. I gave myself another challenge when I decided that I wanted to pursue my second degree at another school, the prestigious Architectural Association School of Architecture. The entrance interview happened during the term of my final academic year, and I had not prepared well. I had unknowingly organised a portfolio that was completely abstract and failed to show material that displayed my technical knowledge. The interviewers were therefore unsure of my capabilities, and decided that for me to be accepted, I had to repeat my third year again. This was not just disappointing, but also challenging to explain to my sponsors. I explained my situation tactfully, and was relieved to continue to receive their financial support to join the prestigious Architectural Association School of Architecture, from which I eventually graduated with my second degree.

After graduation, I started my working years in Singapore to serve my bond to the Housing and Development Board of Singapore. But there was yet another twist to the final chapter of my education journey when the Registrar of the Architectural Association School contacted me and offered me a scholarship to pursue a Masters degree. This meant that I only had to come up with my living expenses.

At that time, this was something very unusual. For me it was a very big deal, because I could never have afforded an education like this. I started to make plans to save up so that I could support myself through the Masters year. And I ended up leaving the country again to complete the 13-month Masters program. As far as my design thinking is concerned, this was one of the key periods that changed my design mindset and methodology. In that program I met my Argentinian tutor, who was more holistic and systems-based in the way he approached issues, rather than designing for function and aesthetics. His perspective was so much broader and, in a way, taught me and gave me amazingly new insights, which were way more than I had learnt previously. It was a different depth of learning and opened my mind completely.

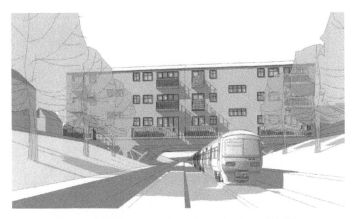

IMAGE: RENDERING OF PROPOSED HOMES OVER TRACKS, HOMES ON BRIDGES, AKA HOTHOB, WHICH WAS A RESEARCH PROJECT PRESENTED AT THE LONDON FESTIVAL OF ARCHITECTURE 2018. THE CONCEPT WAS UNDERPINNED BY THE EXPLORATION OF UN-TAPPED SITES THAT CAN HELP SOLVE LONDON'S HOUSING CRISIS.

Source: DPA

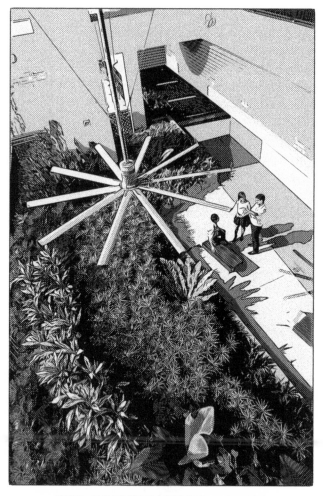

PHOTO: ONE OF MANY GENEROUS SKY GARDENS
WITHIN THE BUILDING CLEANTECH ONE, SINGAPORE.

Source: Suvbana

MY BENEFACTORS

I feel that my life up to now has been a miracle. Had I not taken the initiative to tweak my fate at various moments, things would likely have turned out quite differently. The Vice Principal (1984) at River Valley High School, the Vice Principal (1989) at National Junior College, the Human Resource Manager (scholarship processing, 1993) at HDB, the Registrar (1999) at the AA School of Architecture: they are all my benefactors and unsung heroes. If any of them had taken the stance of "why should I bother," my educational journey and, therefore, my career would have taken a very different course.

I reflect on this nowadays as "the twists and turns of my life." Our journey often leads us to forks in the road, and which path we take makes a small but ultimately big difference to which direction we take. Small but big.

In some ways, this also serves to explain why I ended up being both extremely successful professionally and concurrently chronically and deeply depressed in the years to come.

BECOMING DAD

Many years of working ensued and the next major change occurred for me when my first daughter, Ella, was born. I was just half a year short of turning 40, relatively old for a first-time father, and I recall the emotions and events of Ella's birth as a big change, a big mental rewiring of my previously career-focused mental circuit board.

Holding my baby when she was just born, I recall tears streaming down my face uncontrollably for two hours. I was overwhelmed with emotions. I believe it was at that moment when I felt the first awareness of what I today call meaning and purpose.

Having my first child transformed me. It changed the way I perceived work and the way life was meant to be. It had to be something bigger than pursuing a career, or trying to become famous and established. In 2012, this realisation led me to taking a year off from working, which then resulted in me returning to Singapore, before I returned to London, my current permanent relocation to the UK.

SHARPENING OUR SAWS

Often, it is crucial to step back from what we are busy with, and pause for a moment, to re-assess if our efforts are well invested, and reaping for us deserved results.

Stephen Covey shares in his major work *Seven Habits of Highly Effective Leaders*[4] about working on our mental fitness. I am most fascinated by the chapter titled "Sharpening our Saw." In today's society, it is extremely important that we work on understanding ourselves: our mental well-being, our physical well-being, the state of our happiness, and our mental modalities and mindset. The ability to pause and really get into our mindset is sharpened by our awareness. This is a key step to discovering our unique ability, and then attaining our ambition, followed by our quest to find fulfilment and enjoyment in life. Each of us can be present for ourselves and everyone around us, in many different shapes and forms, and we play many different roles.

When we look at our constant interactions with the external world, we must realise how we are affected internally. Ignoring the internal state leaves residual emotions that can result in a sense of negativity. It is therefore vital for us to look at our environment and how it affects us in all aspects of our being.

*"I HOPE THIS INTRODUCTION HELPS
TO GIVE SOME INSIGHTS INTO HOW TO
APPRECIATE AND USE THIS BOOK.
ITS PURPOSE IS TO ENCOURAGE YOU TO
INVESTIGATE AND TO TAKE A LEAP OF FAITH TO
JOIN THE WHAD MOVEMENT: NOT JUST ACQUIRE
AN AWARENESS OF IT, BUT ALSO TO TAKE SOME
VERY SPECIFIC, DETERMINED STEPS TO TWEAK THE
LIFE AROUND US SO THAT WE CAN THEN
BRING FURTHER JOY AND HAPPINESS TO BOTH
OURSELVES AND THE PEOPLE WHO SURROUND US."*

UP NEXT ...

In the next chapter, I share my unique
approach to health and well-being from the
design and architecture perspective.

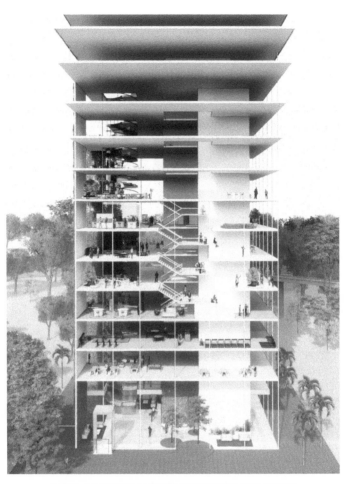

IMAGE: RENDERING OF EXPLORATORY RESEARCH PROJECT
TITLED "WELLSKYSCRAPER", INTENDED TO PROMOTE CONSIDERATIONS OF
WORKPLACES SPECIFICALLY CONCEIVED FOR WELLBEING-INFUSED SPACES,
WITH AN EMPHASIS TO BATTLE INACTIVITY.

Source: Author's own collection

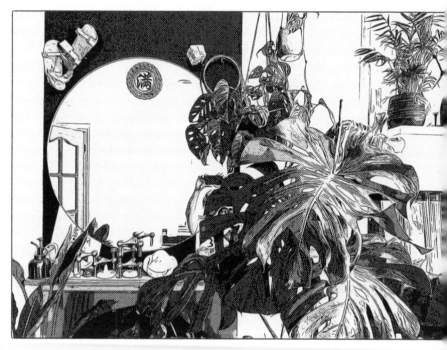

PHOTO: CONTROL OF MATERIAL PALETTE
ALONGSIDE INDOOR PLANTS AT MY OWN HOME.

Source: Author's own collection

CHAPTER 2

THE EUREKA
OF WHAD:

Seeing the Light
I Have to Be

*"A HEALTHY MAN WANTS A THOUSAND THINGS,
A SICK MAN ONLY WANTS ONE."*

CONFUCIUS

How much of our destiny and how much
of our ability to perform is within our own
control? Is there anything with which we
surround ourselves that affects our ability to
manage our own destiny? What can we do to
shape our environment and create spaces that
elevate us to a state of becoming happier and
healthier, both physically and mentally?

This chapter will show you how the physical
environment we dwell in is closely related to
our functional performance as human beings.
How the hardware, which is the environment,
is actually a major influence on the software,
our physical being. Our mental capacity can

be adjusted, to a considerable degree, by the spaces that surround us.

You can do different spatial improvements with any budget, or regardless of budget. We can make our living spaces and our workplaces align with our needs, no matter what kind of environment we face or live in. These spaces can become conducive to empowering ourselves to perform at a higher level, much like how meditation can help a sportsperson achieve higher goals. I will show you what I have learned and gathered over 25 years of my professional practice as an architect.

I will share the lessons I have learnt through hardship, relating back to my own challenges with my mental well-being, and how I have moved through it and grown. I will also articulate how I have instilled in myself the ability to use my technical design knowledge to formulate and enhance a system of using design to generate and create well-being targets to make everyone happier. First, let's debunk some presumptions about designing our spaces.

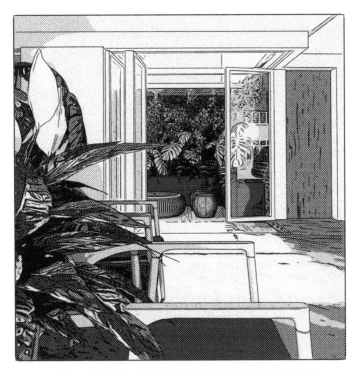

IMAGE: A COMPACT COURTYARD PROPOSED FOR THE EXTENSION
OF A CHIROPRACTOR'S WELL-BEING LIFESTYLE CLINIC.
(LOCATION: NORTH LONDON)

Source: Author's own collection

THREE MYTHS OR MISCONCEPTIONS

These are the three main misconceptions about
happiness and well-being-enabling spaces:

Myth 1:

Happiness and well-being are not influenced by our environment.

Happiness has a lot to do with our physical environment and our surroundings. Our surroundings enhance and facilitate the forming of human relationships, the forming of bonds and the growth of our emotional states.

Happiness is a state of being. Feeling accomplished or being thrilled by physical experiences or the attainment of material objects is, again, not true happiness. Instead, happiness and well-being are very sophisticated states of mind, sometimes transient, and for certain aspects are more deeply ingrained in our subconscious.

Myth 2:

If we are not in a state of unhappiness, then there is nothing we need to do. Because if something is not broken, there is no need to fix it.

This is a false belief or an incorrect understanding, just like the belief that being healthy is the absence of illness. It can be the case that you are without illness, but you are not necessarily healthy. So, similarly, being without unhappiness is not equal to being happy.

Constantly being aware of our inner state also means maintaining a level of mental fitness that enables us to face our daily struggles. That is why it is necessary to create living spaces that help us lead a balanced lifestyle, and feel nurtured and safe.

Myth 3:

Designing or styling your space can only be done by professionally trained people, either interior designers, interior architecture designers or architects.

If you recall your childhood, you might remember building your own tents and play areas with blankets, sheets and furniture. We did this to feel secure and comforted. These self-decorated areas enabled us to be in an elevated or happier state as children engaging in imaginative play.

We can create our own living spaces in a way that comforts us, that gives us a sense of balance.

THREE SIMPLE TRUTHS

Even though nothing is broken, a lot can still be made better. These are three truths that are simple, but often overlooked.

Truth 1:

Each of us can and ought to take ownership of our own environment, feel in control of our own spaces and make changes to enrich our everyday habits and lifestyle.

The most subtle and constant way that we can improve our mental states is to develop better habits, and better habits can be facilitated if we create for ourselves conducive environments.

Truth 2:

Many of these changes and enhancements are within the capacity of any individual. With some basic knowledge and skills, some of these changes are purely logical and simple to execute.

The best design interventions are those that involve small and inexpensive alterations to otherwise conventional but dysfunctional details. It is also important to not focus on following trends, as they will likely not address your particular circumstances and more likely be driven by the commercial agenda of looks and aesthetics alone.

Truth 3:

Even if one is limited by budget, it is still possible to consider many simple and effective adjustments to a space.

Often, the most powerful impact is making small improvements to a space, sometimes making adjustments in small degrees over a period of time, which then help us grow good new habits.

If we keep ignoring minor misconceptions, we start to construct in our minds a more complex version of a false truth. Our brain has the power to reinforce images and beliefs regardless of their truth. It is important to recognise that such false truths can at times become so overwhelmingly sophisticated, and so convincingly real, that we will actually require a major overhaul, much like completely stripping the engine of an old motorcar and redoing everything.

This is the similar to the way we should constantly work on and pay attention to our mental health. The same attention, also, is needed to the way that we deal with the physical environment that surrounds us.

My mental health suffered prolonged damage over a period of 10 years. The COVID lockdown of 2020 exacerbated this condition.

In the middle of the first lockdown I was in the worst state ever, feeling suicidal. Many of the reflections that I've gathered and included in this book are the result of awakening from that nightmare.

Recovering from such a deeply troubled mental space required that I develop a perspective of life that is more compassionate and empathetic of my immediate environment.

I began to explore the idea that many simple and budget-friendly changes can be made to a space during my mental health recovery. Having always felt a subconscious need to design my space with certain colours and materials, I often wondered why. I realised around this time that it gave me a sense of comfort, and this sense stabilised as I began to understand more about the powerful force transmitted by our surroundings through our senses, and the way it is almost always affects us internally.

Here is one such study that gives us a deeper insight into this aspect.

PROJECT STAIRWELL[5]

Inactivity is the fourth worst killer,[6] as classified by the World Health Organization. This unfortunate consequence of our modern sedentary lifestyle affects us not only physically, but to a large extent mentally, too.

Project *stairWELL* was conceived and executed over a period of nearly a year in Singapore. It was government-funded research supported by a Good Design Research grant from the Design Singapore Council. We inserted physical interventions into an existing staircase within the work environment of the Singapore media company, MediaCorp, to investigate how slight tweaks to the existing space might increase the use of the staircase between two floors, and dissuade the occupants from choosing the lift.

Principally, the project attempted to address how people could increase the frequency of movement in their work environment. It was an in-depth study with the aim to enhance both physical and mental well-being through becoming more active at the workplace.

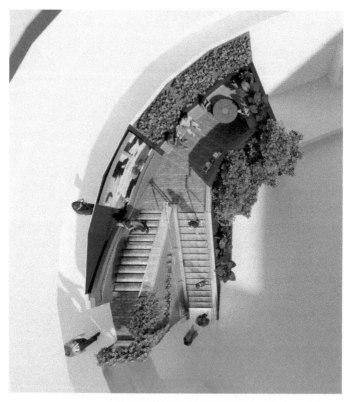

DRAWING: ILLUSTRATION SHOWING THE PROPOSAL OF A MULTI-FUNCTIONAL STAIRCASE WITHIN A WORKPLACE ATRIUM SETTING.

Source: Author's own collection

This research work is instrumental in demonstrating that subtle tweaks to an uninteresting architectural circulation device can instigate rather drastic changes to our movement patterns. Our study demonstrated that increased use of the stairs instead of the lift was achievable through creative treatments such as adding of plants and imagery that evoke mental associations Amongst the various interventions we carried out, adding pictorial imagery resulted in an increase of the trips made at the stairs to as much as almost 3 times.

With the calories burnt when climbing up four floors at the workspace, one only has to make six of such trips between work tasks throughout the day to achieve the same effect as taking a deliberate 10 min brisk exercise walk of a mile. Also, this kind of smaller bursts of movements are far more achievement in habit forming than initiating a more drastic exercise routine.

Many minor adjustments to the spaces surrounding us can change the way we see ourselves, the way we see the people around us and the manner in which we undertake our daily activities.

Elements within a building can be adjusted to moderate our intuitive patterns of using them. In my work I have been fascinated with how interstitial and connecting spaces, such as corridors and stairs, are too often overlooked. I see a lot of potential in addressing how we move and interact with such circulatory spaces to impact everyday habits. It is not just the zones where we spend the most time that can make a difference. The routes and gaps in between them do too, but these less glamorous spaces have not been given enough attention.

The pandemic opened our eyes to how health is wealth. In the US alone, prescriptions for psychiatric medication went up 34% in 2020 due to the influence of the COVID-19 pandemic. One can have great financial wealth but it does not necessarily give us a healthy self. Anyone is as equally vulnerable to threats to their health as an unhoused person sleeping on the streets. COVID-19 and my own mental health battle called to me to address the way design and architecture can positively impact our overall health and well-being.

YOUR SPACE AND YOU

Wherever you are, and whatever space you are in, elements of our environment interface with our physical body as well as with our mental states. Understanding how our senses and our sensory intuition are related to the spaces that we exist in, the environments where we spend time, is crucial. It is necessary to understand our own preferences, our own intuitive knowledge of materiality and textures, and other physical aspects of how a space or an environment is defined.

In this book, we start to look at an individual's unique palette of materiality. This includes colours, textures, tactile elements, and the way the physical space interacts with the external environment. One of the insights we want to achieve for ourselves here, is to gain an understanding of the functional spaces.

Traditionally, we tend to understand that a space serves a physical activity and a function. But what is more intriguing is to understand that an activity or function is inherently an aspect of how we exist in the universe.

For example, the dining space has, for most, the primary function of providing a space or a location for the act of eating. However, the act of eating is merely a technical function, whilst the process and experience of having a meal together, I would argue, is the true primary function. And this function is about spending time either by yourself, enjoying a meal, or with others, having conversations with members of your family or people that you care about. This is the core purpose your dining or eating space is meant to really serve, enhancing our well-being and happiness.

The evolution of our human species is innate to our need to create a certain kind of space for safety. Some of the insights I share are grounded in research in neuroscience, anthropology and archaeology. The fact is that we are fundamentally modern cavemen, hardwired to process stimuli in a way that we have an initial instinctive gut feel, leading us to a "fight, flight or freeze" response. These are underlying responses that make it difficult to react to the challenges of today. Our personal spaces, whether our homes or our offices, are where we can find solace, heal our wounds and protect ourselves from the harsh elements of our stress packed day. How we design these spaces reflects our need to come home to being ourselves.

Another innate human need is the desire to belong to a group. From the perspective of evolution theory, this gives us the security and safety we need for survival and protection from danger. This is something that is deeply embedded in our brain. We have evolved into beings that process our environments in this way. From this comes a need for belonging, which reflects our tribal human history. The reason why we as a species have continued to exist is because we have successfully hard-wired our instincts for survival and self-preservation.

We have to understand ourselves and be able to give attention to self-care and self-love so that we can have a positive attitude to our own existence. By doing so, we allow ourselves to become effective members of a larger group. As we connect the dots of our experiences in life, in the same way that all of us did from my childhood experiences to adulthood, we get closer to understanding how our brain and how our sense of curiosity functions.

Humans are always inquisitive and want to learn something new. This is due to our natural desire to develop our skills and capabilities. When expanded more broadly, it is also about creating a better situation for the entity that is larger than us as an individual: for example, our family unit, our community, the society and, ultimately, the world.

That we constantly strive to create a better world requires more than an intention: it also depends heavily on our mental fitness. Not many people will negate or dispute that. However, we have grown up with the false logic that because we have become adults, we have acquired more and more knowledge and skills, so much so that we can learn less and less. This is when I recall the importance of the Don't Know, Don't Know[7] principle, the DKDK quadrant of this mental mind map, which will be discussed in more detail in the next chapter.

What this DKDK idea deals with is extremely basic and at the same time it is important. As we get older, we should expand our awareness and be humble enough to accept that there are things we are not aware that we do not know.

Youth is a time of being open to new ways of looking at the world. DKDK is accepting that we simply do not know everything. Instead of putting our heads in the sand and refuse to engage with this truth, I urge that we be as humble as we can, which opens our minds to new possibilities in our ever-evolving world.

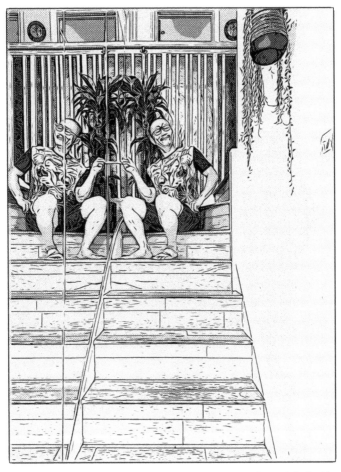

PHOTO: THE USE OF BASIC BUT INNOVATIVE DESIGN TECHNIQUES SUCH AS MIRRORS AT THE RIGHT PLACES CAN HELP CREATE THE ILLUSION OF SPACE.

In this book, I offer actionable strategies and highlight a few key spaces within the home environment which are critical elements of our modern everyday living. We might not have given them full attention or exercised care and love in the way that we curate these spaces so that they actually shape us, and in a way affect our inner world.

When we shape our environments, our environments shape us. I will give you insights and suggestions as to ideas on how you can develop some techniques and implement some small tweaks to a few key spaces in your home as well as ideas for your workplace. I will expand on what ways the WHAD movement is meant to serve ourselves, our families, and humanity. The process of taking small actions can lead to big changes in our lives. It is my hope that this movement, via the sheer existence of this small book, could start us on a much bigger journey. Small but big.

UP NEXT ...

In the next chapter, we discuss the way we see knowledge as a quest that is perpetually using the concept of Don't Know Don't Know.

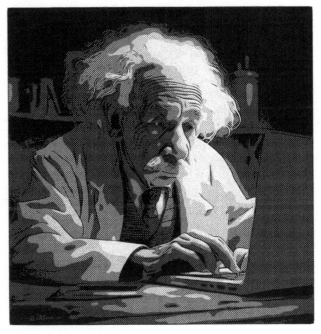

IMAGE: IF EINSTEIN HAD ADDITIONAL TECHNOLOGY TO ASSIST HIS
INVESTIGATIONS, WHAT WOULD HIS CORE QUEST BE ABOUT TODAY?

Source: Rendering by author, generated by AI using Midjourney

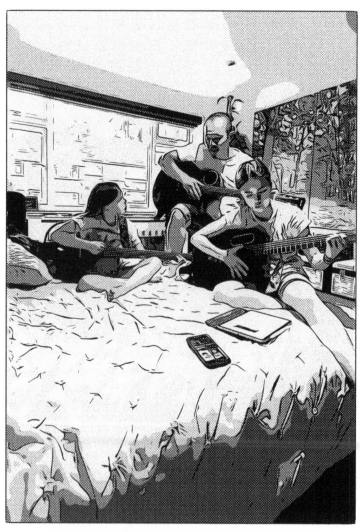

PHOTO: TIME WELL SPENT. WHEN MOMENTS BECOME REGISTERED
AS DISTINCTIVE CHAPTERS OF YOUR EXPERIENCE DATABANK.

CHAPTER 3

CURIOSITY AND COMPETENCE:

Don't Know Don't Know aka DKDK

"WE NOW ACCEPT THE FACT THAT LEARNING IS A LIFELONG PROCESS OF KEEPING ABREAST OF CHANGE. AND THE MOST PRESSING TASK IS TO TEACH PEOPLE HOW TO LEARN."

PETER DRUCKER

Today's world is extremely fast-paced. Never have we lived in a society in which technology advances at such a phenomenal rate. While humanity becomes increasingly superior, equally we feel challenged every single day. Importantly, we must understand that we need to keep our minds open to new ideas, because it is this willingness to absorb new things and to process new situations that allows us to keep up.

How many times have you been in a conversation and offered a well-meaning suggestion, or a piece of advice, and received the response,

"I know, I know" even before you finished your sentence?

Eight out of Ten people I have come across behave in exactly this way, and they are not open to learning because they are almost too confident that they already know anything and everything that needs to be learned. They are resistant to learning anything new. Humility is essential to learning and being open to new ideas.

One of the traits that I try to teach myself which does not come naturally to me (I admit I do have to make quite a bit of effort), is to not be fixated on what I already know. Instead, I try to be completely intrigued and always eager to learn and appreciative of what I do not know. Anyone who is too confident and assumes that they already know everything that needs to be known is, in an ironic way, robbing themselves of the opportunity to engage with greater things to come.

This chapter is as much about self-confidence as it is about managing our own humility and recognising our need to keep an open mind. Keeping our overconfidence in check and using it positively and constructively is extremely important. Very little is discussed about the coexistence of confidence and humility. While these two things might seem to be opposites, it is important to recognise that they do indeed coexist, and this awareness is critically important for personal growth. We often deprive ourselves of fantastic insights and knowledge when we shield and distance ourselves with the egoistical protection of, "I already know it all."

By the end of this chapter, you will see how our awareness of what we perceive around us belongs in one of three of the four quadrants. When we are interested to unlock the fourth quadrant - DKDK (i.e. don't know, don't know) - we unlock a vast, often unrecognised possibility to grow, thrive, play and explore.

The principle of DKDK is rooted in philosophy. It is exactly how our brain functions, and not just marketing or positive-thinking jargon.

By becoming aware of our unconscious incompetence, which is the more academic term for DKDK, we can expand very effectively the knowledge and experience in all the other three quadrants. When we know that we do not know something, we increase our realm of conscious competence, which is the quadrant of what we know, we know.

In this context, I would love to share the behaviour of children, who are the most avid and engaged participants within our environment. In my view, it is because young children are willing (and quite happy) to fail, and through failing, they learn.

NAIVETY IS GOLDEN

Have you ever wondered how children learn so much within such a short span of time? Is it their sheer exposure to new knowledge, new information and new environments, or is it the sponge-like qualities of their minds and their huge desire to just take everything in? I guess the right answer is probably both, but as we grow up to become adults, we often lose the second part of this equation.

What motivates the child is their thirst for information and knowledge, and this thirst is powered by naivety and the lack of fear of embarrassment. As children grow, their natural confidence becomes eroded by our culture's disease of, "Don't show others you don't know, because they will laugh at you. They will ridicule you. They will look down on you." Where did this come from?

Being vulnerable and being naive, especially as an adult, is frowned upon. The adults with whom we grew up - our parents and teachers - set an example for us and they themselves were instilled with this same belief that showing yourself to be ignorant is embarrassing or humiliating. This is another example of how we pass on beliefs that are not just far from, but are almost the direct opposite of, real truth.

	Know (K)	don't know (DK)
Know (K)	**KK** **[Assumptions]**	**KDK** **[Gaps]**
don't know (DK)	**DKK** **[Tacit Knowledge]**	**DKDK** **[Blind Spots or Discoveries]**

DIAGRAM: KK+DKK+KDK+DKDK.

Our association with the world falls into four quadrants and I will illustrate it using the above diagram.

Firstly, there is the "know know" quadrant, also known as **KK**. The **KK** quadrant encompasses the information, knowledge and experience that we have learned. We are fully cognisant that we understand this information or possess these skills. This might include academic knowledge and information, the way we operate a piece of equipment, or even daily habits and life skills, like how to brush our teeth. We are aware that we know and we are fully happy with the fact that we know what we know.

Secondly, there is the "know don't know" (KDK) quadrant. This includes the things surrounding us in our lives that we know we don't know. For example, how does one power up a magnificent metallic steel construction, such as a rocket, with enough power to pierce the atmosphere and travel into space? Unless we are aeronautical engineers or scientists, we are aware that we don't know how to make this happen, and that we are perfectly okay with not knowing.

There are also functions happening around and within us that we are not aware that we know. For example, the brain is fully capable of coordinating the beating of the heart and synchronising it with the intake and the expelling of air through our noses and mouths and the functioning of the lungs. The brain is fully capable of knowing how it works. We might not spend time thinking about it, but the fact is our human body is capable of doing it. Unless we are medically trained or have expertise, we cannot understand the exact details. So, this falls into the category of something we do not know that we know, or **DKK**.

Finally, there are the many things that we don't know we don't know, or **DKDK**. If you close your eyes and think back on today, yesterday, or last week you might recall something which, if you are truly honest with yourself, you were not even aware that you did not know. Assuming your mind was open enough to pay attention to it, you realise that there was something that you were not aware of previously, and you were not even aware that this was something that you did not know before. With this newfound awareness, you can change your environment to suit your needs.

This is an example of a mindset change. The ability to think about changes will help you to think about how adjustments to your environment can impact your personal life as well as those surrounding you.

Here, we are going to talk about techniques to understand this DKDK concept so we can begin to apply it to our lives. This can also give us clarity to make sense of things that we might not be able to figure out. These could be spatial techniques, or they could be action plans relating to how we organise the space around us. Say, for example, you are currently working in a room where there is a lot of clutter, with piles of papers and maybe even stacks of half-read books. By making an adjustment through spring-cleaning, you are effectively clearing the clutter not just physically, but also in your mind space. Mentally, the brain feels lighter and you create more space for the brain to function and become more lucid. It has the freedom to exercise its creativity and productivity more effectively. Less clutter, more clarity.

I had a WhatsApp conversation with my mother during the pandemic lockdown in 2020. We were talking about the acquisition of knowledge and the way that we simply know so little. I said, "The dumbest person is the guy who keeps saying, 'I know, I know,' and the cleverest person is the one who genuinely believes they know very little and has an insatiable, or perhaps even aggressive, appetite to listen to and learn from others. This is that fire and that hunger to fuel the DKDK quadrant."

My mother encouraged me to exercise wisdom from this insight and told me that being inquisitive and humble is a golden trait. Having read about neuroscience and getting glimpses of how our behaviours can be reprogrammed, such as research findings about neuroplasticity,[8] I was extremely excited and intrigued.

HEALTH THROUGH EXERCISE, OR THROUGH MIND?

It was a magic, "Aha!" moment when I read about the experiment that Dr Ellen Langer[9] and her colleague conducted on hotel assistants.

There were two groups of hotel assistants whose daily tasks included cleaning the rooms, changing bedsheets and doing a number of other physical tasks as part of their work routine. Of course, the research was done without revealing to the two groups what was being measured. They were just given an appraisal of what activities they did, with one group being given an insight into how many calories their daily work was consuming. The staff members were told that the amount of physical work they were doing was equal to a two-hour gym workout. Several weeks later, when all the participants were revisited, those who were given this information had appreciable improvements to their physical health, without their knowing. This intriguing research exposed how powerful the mind is, and how the awareness of outcomes leads us, even in our physical bodies, to respond in ways that we were not previously capable of. Reading this opened up my mind to how the learnings from neuroscience can be combined with my work.

LEARNING FROM THE DEEP SELF

Another example is from brain expert Jim Kwik.[10] His Mindvalley course, titled "Superpowers of the Brain," unlocked my mind and the way that I see things, and that led to the beginnings of the DKDK concept.

What the course triggered me to do was to think deeply and realise that many things that we might normally consider impossible are in fact rather plausible. Jim is able to accomplish fascinating tasks through the way he taps into the maximum potential of the brain. In fact, the word "impossible," broken down, is spelt I-M-possible. This gave me the ability and the courage to rebrand and reinvent myself, to think of myself as someone who can endeavour to do much more than I had before until then.

Being trained as an architect and having the skills to design spaces and architecture of all scales, my interest was to embrace my newly acquired knowledge and combine it with design as a way to improve lives. I want to motivate people to have an inquisitive nature and be childlike. We should all become as naive and be as curious as the youngest infant. This is how we can become aligned to truly work on our own well-being. To benefit fully from this learning, you must deliberately expose yourself to the awareness that almost everyone around you knows something that you do not. I truly believe this is not far from the truth at all.

We must be on a relentless quest for information and be completely open to new ideas. Being uncomfortable is the best challenge we can gift to ourselves because then we learn and grow to become comfortable with being uncomfortable. This can help us discover our own potential to navigate a fast-changing world.

For example, we might start conversations by saying, "Can you tell me something about you that I don't know?" Our inquisitive nature leads us to try to understand each other. The willingness to learn more about what the other person knows will uplift us to a different level.

THE BOTTOM LINE

In today's world where information and knowledge are easily available, it is neither plausible nor necessary to lay claim to being a person who knows-it-all. The attitude of a humble learner with huge passion and desire to soak in everything that we come close to is a much more productive philosophy and approach to living. This will yield more positive motivations and raise the bar of our own everyday mental well-being.

One of the things that I encourage everyone to do is imagine yourself at three years old and list down three things that you then had no awareness of. This is an example of DKDK. For example, we did not realise that advertisements were the source of income for newspapers and magazines. And that a wide readership would, in turn, attract advertisers in what seems to be a circular economy logic. At some point between the age of three and now, the DKDK turned into one of the other three categories. This exercise allows and our minds to entertain the possibility of further DKDKs. In consciously engaging with the unknown in this way, the positive process continues.

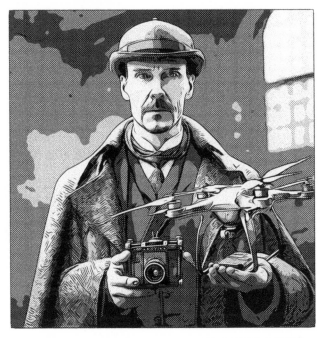

IMAGE: SHERLOCK HOLMES WITH TODAY'S NEWER TECHNOLOGIES.

Source: Author, image generated using AI technology Midjourney

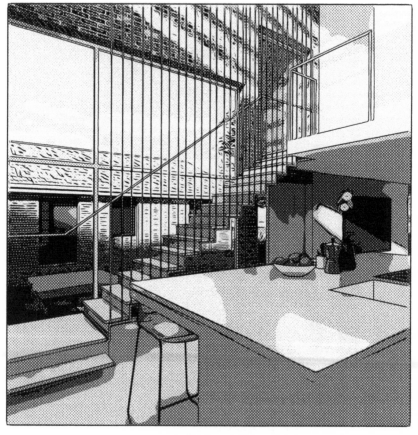

IMAGE: THE CENTRAL SPACE (HEART) OF A PROPOSED COMPACT HOME
PROJECT LOCATED AT NORTH LONDON, UK.

Source: Author's own collection

CHAPTER 4

SIX SENSES

"OUR CREATOR HAS GIVEN US FIVE SENSES TO HELP US SURVIVE THREATS FROM THE EXTERNAL WORLD, AND A SIXTH SENSE, OUR HEALING SYSTEM, TO HELP US SURVIVE INTERNAL THREATS."

BERNIE SIEGEL

Have you ever experienced a sense of unease or discomfort when you enter a café, or a home, or just a space that you came across when you were out walking? On the contrary, have you ever felt a sense of joy and calm in a certain environment? This feeling is more innate and inbuilt than we realise. You experience this through your senses - feel it in your body - before your mind can process it.

We are wired this way. Our antenna is constantly monitoring our external environment, even when our mind is occupied. Our existence and awareness of being in the present is managed by our very powerful central processing unit, the human brain. The way the brain functions, similar to a computer, is through electronic impulses: literally, electrical neuro charges call synapses.[11]

Everything we recognise - whether by sight, touch, smell, taste, sound or by instinct - is processed via brainwaves, also sometimes described as vibrations. The super powerful computers that we are born with, located between our ears, i.e. our brains, are the means by which we evaluate the world that we live in. All the other means, such as our senses, are all its important supporting conduits.

By the end of this chapter, you will understand how aspects of our environment connect within and tap our senses to respond positively or negatively, although most of the time we might not be paying attention to this. You will understand the neural concept of negative bias and the power it has over our subtle reactions (most of which we do not make a deliberate decision about), specifically in relation to space or places. You will also understand how easy and important it can be to create changes in the spaces you live or work in. Making such adjustments can help you function better and will increase your well-being.

Our ability to conjure positive emotions as well as our inability to block out negativity has been studied in the last two or three decades by the world's top neuroscientists.

For example, when we slide our finger across an edge of furniture that is sharp, our instincts tell us there is a chance we might be injured. This awareness has been studied and proven to be more effectively recalled at the next occurrence. A positive experience of curved, blunt furniture edges does not leave such a deep imprint in our memory banks.

I am bringing into the discussion concepts such as neuroplasticity reminding ourselves that our brain and physical body are connected inexorably, sending information both ways.

The underpinning story for evolution is the primary motivation for survival: enabling the continued existence of our species. Simply put, we have to protect ourselves from danger and not get killed, as well as procreate to birth the next generation.

As babies, our notion of the world around us is amazingly open. From our first weeks of life, we get messages from the facial expressions of everyone around us, to guide our behaviour and approach to the world. These messages teach us life skills, the ability (somewhat) to be safe from harm, and to behave appropriately. However, this aspect of what we learn is a human construct; this definition of appropriate (or safe) depends on the definition of a person or persons, usually the parents, based on their own upbringing and interpretations. The rules that are created to guide such existence are quite different from scientific laws like gravity or the workings of oxygen in our bloodstream. Several thought leaders[12] call this human-engineered set of rules our culture-scape, which we internalise as the rules of society and the world.

Our perception of the world is also deeply encoded with our past experiences and memories that construct our mental model. What we do not question enough is whether these mental constructs and causal logics truly make sense at all.

WELL-BEING STANDARDS TO CERTIFY SPACES AND BUILDINGS

According to the International Well-being Institute,[13] the principles of a well-certified building hinge on numerous factors, each of which directly or indirectly addresses the core functions of the human body's six senses.

SIGHT

Our eyes allow us to take in information by light. This information is then sent to the brain and processed in the form of images. Light consists of different wavelengths, each of which has, through our evolution, triggered different responses in our brains. This necessitates a brief mentioning of the topic of circadian rhythm.

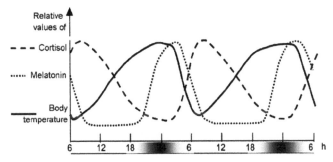

DIAGRAM: CYCLIC VARIATION OF TEMPERATURE, MELATONIN AND CORTISOL IN HUMANS OVER TWO 24 HR CYCLES.[14]

Located at the rear of our eyes is the organ that receives the signal of the amount and type of light that enters our eyes, and this information is transmitted to our brain.[15] Since the dawn of time, humans and other animals have been used to the daily change from day to night and night to day. Once the sun sets the light from the sky loses its natural wavelength of the blue spectrum. The human body can detect this and as a hard-wired response, reduce its charge of cortisol, concocting instead the dosage of melatonin. Scientists have proven that melatonin is released by the brain for us to get ready for rest, and it is directly linked to a good night's sleep.[16]

When humans created artificial light, we created a problem for ourselves. Artificial light, especially that comprising the blue spectrum, is the core reason why there is a sleep problem in today's societies. Current technology is changing the way we use artificial lighting, to either minimise its use, or by tweaking its wavelength compositions accordingly. By using the correct lighting, we can simulate the natural way that daylight (or the lack of it) works, in order for us to ready our bodies to rest and be recharged for the next day.

TOUCH

When it comes to the sense of touch, we are innately in tune with the elements of nature.

When I feel stressed, I take a few moments to walk in my garden barefoot. There is something magical about our feet touching the ground, feeling the earth and the grass, or the way that we glide our fingertips across wood or feel the rippling movements of water. Our belonging to the natural world is evident in the positive feelings we get when we feel the earth and sand between our toes. Being without shoes lets us engage with the ground in a more primitive, and more natural way.

As human beings, we feel instinctively grounded. We embrace and form a connection with the soil or the ground that we walk on. It has only been in recent times that we exist in environments built of metal and glass. Yes, they have not been always there: we created them. This is not to say that metal and glass are damaging or in contradiction to the betterment of mankind: rather, we should get closer to nature and understand why nature has a different (logical) offering.

Nature conjures up feelings about the existence of an environment prior to our own. The combination of nature with nurture is important for us to decipher. By taking the effort to immerse in nature through direct intimate contact, we communicate on a deep level with the world that surrounds us. This, in turn, allows us to learn about the ability of touch to enhance our positive emotions.

SOUND

Where I am sitting now is adjacent to the brook near my home. The constant flow of water as ambient noise is almost a melodious backdrop of music that can elevate a sense of well-being. White noise from nature can be calming background music.

We have all heard that an unborn child in its mother's womb is already listening to sounds and becoming familiar with voices, especially its mother's. The auditory sense is the first medium of informed awareness that develops in us human beings.[17]

Another sensorial aspect of us as human beings is the way that sound can trigger different emotions and memories. The fact that absolute silence is uncomfortable makes us aware that sound plays a huge part in our appreciation of any environment. In fact, scientific experiments have proven that there is increased comfort and heightened sense of well-being when we are in an environment where sound is masked,[18] muffling the conversations we do not want to hear. This is the reason why we have ambient music in many shopping centres. As a design intervention, introducing sounds created by flowing water in workplaces improves employees' concentration and experience of the workplace.

SMELL AND TASTE

Smell and taste are also important senses which detect whether our environment is favourable to us or not. Our sense of smell can immediately tell us if something is dangerous. When we eat, we are attracted to the food's aroma first, causing our mouths to water. Taste is the secondary sense through which we can understand the food's sweetness, sourness, bitterness and saltiness before we ingest it.

Recent scientific experiments have proven that taste is greatly influenced by smell, because of what researchers call retro nasal perception.[19] One such example which uses this finding is a relatively new and very successful water bottle product from which one drinks plain water. Named "Air-up,"[20] the water bottle hacks the brain's perception so that the water is perceived to have a taste. This is done by a small device which emits a small that is, in turn, picked up by the olfactory system. In perceiving the scent, we are almost convinced that there is a flavour to the water. Many people dislike drinking water, and this is one of the reasons why this product is, in my opinion, a fabulous innovation.

SIXTH SENSE

So far, the five most straightforward senses have been discussed. What about the sixth?

Some call this sixth sense intuition, while others refer to it as gut feel. This sixth sense is what a cat or dog gears up with in anticipation of its owners coming home. My neighbour across the road, who can see my bedroom window, recently told me that they have on numerous occasions observed my dog, Roxie, appear at the window a few minutes before my car appears. Such stories are not rare, with pets positioning themselves at the doorway moments before the owners arrive home.

This ability to sense what is about to happen is why animals seek shelter or refuge before imminent danger or sudden changes in weather conditions. I believe that this is linked to a gift of intuition grown (or cultivated) throughout evolution. I subscribe to the belief that human beings have it, too, but that we have - because of our rational brain's active decisions - shut it down or at least blocked it out. Might this function that we have turned off be switched back on? To some extent, we have to work on re-wiring our impulses to trust our gut instincts a little more.

THE REPTILIAN BRAIN
AND NEGATIVE BIAS

The first part of the human brain that evolved was the reptilian brain: that part which is the immediate continuation of the spinal cord. This part of the brain oversees the "fight or flight" response. At the early stages of human evolution, there was no need for more sophisticated brain processes; instead, the fight or flight response was pure intuition, or gut feel, with which we sense when the environment is dangerous. It is important to reiterate that this "fight or flight" instinct is spontaneous.

Even now our reactions, and the way that we follow them up with physical actions, are greatly influenced by this fight or flight response.

In order for humans to continue to survive and protect ourselves, our brains learned early to register anything that is negative and, most importantly, what has the potential to cause us physical harm. Recall the first time when, as a child, you cut yourself with something sharp or burned yourself with something hot. You remember it, and it becomes deep awareness; you do not need to note it down, and you almost certainly never repeat that mistake again because such knowledge of potential harm or danger is extremely important. This intuition is linked to what I am about to discuss here, which is the way our brain recognises negative bias.

This instinctive bias is ingrained and deeply embedded in our mental circuit board. Negative bias is the ability to recognize and remember negative moments or negative experiences. This bias is not something the human brain is able to consciously manage to have or not have. One of the easier to understand examples of it is when your fingertips feel something sharp. You get hurt, but the reality is that in future, even without running your fingertips across something sharp, the visual recognition and awareness that an item looks sharp already sends impulses to your brain for you to restrain yourself. These impulses come from the negative bias embedded in your DNA and in the way your brain works. This understanding applies even to our everyday experiences, such as arguments and disagreements between people.

For those of you who have a spouse or a life partner, think how easy is it to remember the pleasurable moments as compared to the fights and the arguments. I bet the fights and the arguments are easier and more deeply ingrained in your memory, and you remember more specific details about them than the positive experiences.

SUBCONSCIOUS GEOMETRY
PREFERENCE EXPERIMENT

Findings in the field of neuroscience have recently shown that something as simple as geometric shapes can stimulate neural impulses similar to a threat response. These impulses, though not severe, have measurable effects from the baseline. This is much like putting our muscles under perpetual mild stress and not allowing any respite: our muscles eventually become permanently deprived of recovery and less able to attain good performance.[21]

Conversely, the use of geometric shapes either simulating what is visible in nature, or echoing the fractal-based algorithms of nature's growth logic, can instil a perpetual positive impact on our mental well-being.[22]

HANDCRAFTED FURNITURE POLL:
SHARP OR CURVED EDGES?

In recent years, I began working on a range of handcrafted birch ply furniture. As an experiment, I detailed two different approaches to the edges and corners of the same stool. I then asked people online, using a poll, which version of the edge detail they instinctively preferred. The findings were interesting.

Approximately 80% of the respondents preferred the curved option, and most commented that this stool looked more comfortable and calming than the more precise (sharper-edged) alternative. Although there are not many scientific findings published yet, I am inclined to believe that there is a close relationship between our choice of less "dangerous" edges and corners, and our subconscious preference to avoid danger. We choose safety and calm, rather than danger and anxiety.[23]

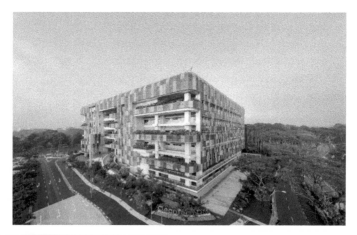

PHOTO: CLEANTECH ONE BUILDING, SINGAPORE.
Source: Suvbana

These instinctive preferences are hardwired in our reptilian brains, the base logic of our bodies' central processing units, which evolved from our caveman times.

CURVED EDGED BUILDING

This same smooth surface treatment was deployed on a building I conceived in 2009-10 (See Photo: Cleantech One Building, Singapore). As the principal designer, I led a team to conceive this urban infrastructure that promotes research lab spaces. To conceal the bulk of the rather large building, which measured almost 50m on each side, we adopted a technique that smoothed the sides using curved chamfered corners. Even at this urban scale, the approach was effective at cushioning the hardness of a sizeable insertion into a (then) rather natural zone of western Singapore. Although we have not been able to carry out research to determine the response to the building, in the years since it was completed I have received a lot of positive feedback that mentioned the unexplained sense of softness and harmony the external treatment allowed observers to feel.

IMAGE: CHAMFERED CORNERS AND EDGES OF BUILDING (CTO).

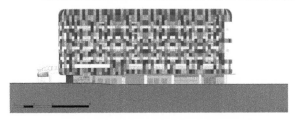

DRAWING: ELEVATION OF THE CHAMFERED CUBE DESIGN FOR CLEANTECH ONE.

Source: Author's own collection

These two examples of differing scales, one of a piece of furniture and the other a large urban building, serve as examples of how there is a sixth sense that we possess in addition to the others that we can describe much more easily.

We unconsciously register so much about negative experiences. It takes no real effort for us to remember not to go near a particular object that caused us harm in the past. The brain is most careful to remember harm. This negative bias is sometimes unproductive, because the brain remembers unpleasant and uncomfortable instances more deeply than happier incidents. What we have to recognize, therefore, is that there is a much stronger negative bias than there is any positive bias. In fact, there is no positive bias, as positive experiences need to be much more deliberately and deeply registered to be long-lasting.

OUR SIX SENSES HELP US CONNECT WITH OUR ENVIRONMENT

All six senses come together to form the way we perceive spaces, experiences and our interactions with one another. It is important for us to understand these fundamental concepts before we can work on delivering the conditions that will give us improved well-being and happiness.

How do our six senses relate to our interfacing with our environment? Which elements in everyday spaces do we use our senses to pay more attention to?

There is a myriad of attributes of our environment that can affect its potential for enhancing wellbeing for us as users of these spaces.

Here, we start to look at just the three aspects that are the easiest to act upon. Within our everyday living environments, these are:-

1. AIR QUALITY

A research experiment relating to how air quality affects our cognitive function was carried out at Berkeley Lab[24] more than 10 years ago.

How absurd for us to lock up the best brains in a meeting rooms for numerous hours drinking coffee

In the experiment, the participants were tested on their mental processing abilities within environments that had levels of carbon dioxide that are reasonably possible at homes or workplaces when air quality is not paid enough attention to. The research produced evidence to explain how high levels of carbon dioxide concentration can degrade the human cognitive functions of taking initiative and strategic thinking, close to the level of being dysfunctional.

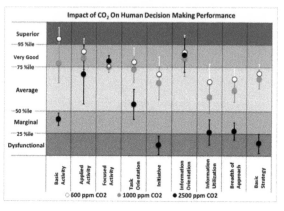

DIAGRAM: CHART SHOWING THE VARIOUS EFFECTS
OF COGNITIVE PROCESSING ALONGSIDE
CO2 CONCENTRATION CATEGORIES.

This tends to happen in many modern workplaces where we are trying to solve complicated problems. The reality is we are not giving ourselves the best chance of good performance due to poor indoor air quality arising from the sheer increase of carbon dioxide within a confined and poorly ventilated space.

This scientific experiment proved that carbon dioxide has damaging effects on brain function, particularly on problem solving, not to mention any good chance of creativity.

2. HYDRATION

The Well Institute recommends a daily consumption of 3.7 litres of water for a grown man and 2.7 litres of water for a woman.[25] However, a recent study carried out in the US revealed that only about 13% of all grown adults there consumed these recommended quantities.

It is commonly known that the human body comprises between 60-70% of water in weight ratio. According to most scientific journals, the brain and heart are composed of 73% water, and the lungs are about 83% water. The skin contains 64% water, muscles and kidneys are 79%, and even our bones are made up of 31% water.[26]

Despite these well published statistics, our habits nowadays in sustaining our hydration levels has probably never been worse. We are distracted and have begun to de-prioritise this basic necessity for our bodies to function.

Instead of relying on ourselves counting glasses of water we drink, I have found that it makes more sense to always have within our reach water bottles of known capacities which will help us become more aware of our hydration habits. At least for myself, this has helped me to grow the habit of drinking enough.

3. SLEEP HYGIENE

The third aspect of our daily pattern that needs improvement is to become aware of the importance of circadian rhythms to our sleep.[27,28]

Sleep hygiene has, in more recent years, become important because of our increasingly hectic lifestyles, coupled with the emergence of advanced technology. How often do we sit in bed using a technological device, either a phone or a tablet? We need to work on having more discipline around our technology and screen use to promote good sleeping habits which will enhance our sleep cycles.

INTERFACING WITH ENVIRONMENT

For all of these three aspects to work optimally, we should consider small changes which can reap big benefits in our lives. If we are open-minded and curious enough, we can embrace that we need to learn, thereby keeping ourselves up to date with new knowledge and methodologies for living better lives.

Our world can be defined as everything that immediately surrounds us. By focusing on the immediate environment that we interface with, and being cognisant of the properties of it that affect us, we can take advantage of a range of opportunities for us to self-adjust.

So, for example, we might look at the ventilation, colours, lighting, materials, and the arrangement of smells, textures and tastes in order for us to have more positive experiences. These changes need not be extreme. They can be subtle and might in fact be quite minor. Although such changes are seemingly trivial and easy, the real impact can very quickly manifest into greater well-being and happiness.

TRY THIS OUT

Choose three of the six senses. Look around at your immediate environment, preferably your home, and try to decipher whether there are aspects of this space that you either like or you do not like. Consider your feelings about these aspects when you consider how your senses respond to them. Write these details, and your responses, in a journal and be articulate about how your brain is processing these considerations.

Remember, every single aspect of the space that we interact with unknowingly effects our well-being.

UP NEXT ...

In the next chapter I will share how materials and the physical existence of objects, things that you can hold and touch, can relate to the senses and how we interact with them. There is a recipe for concocting good emotions and sensibilities, which we will also address.

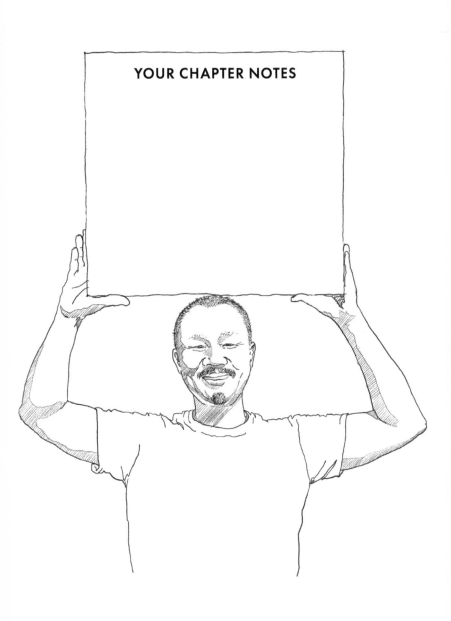

YOUR CHAPTER NOTES

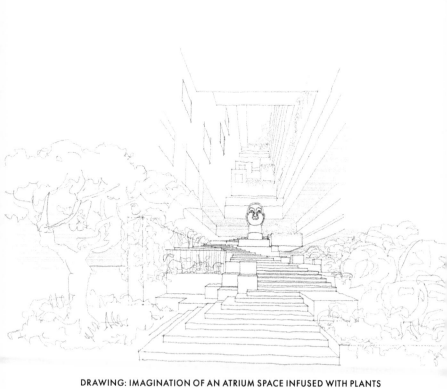

DRAWING: IMAGINATION OF AN ATRIUM SPACE INFUSED WITH PLANTS
AND EXPOSED TO NATURAL LIGHT.

CHAPTER 5

THE POWER OF MATERIALITY:

Nuances and Magic
Ingredients in Our
Natural World

"STUDY NATURE, LOVE NATURE, STAY CLOSE TO NATURE. IT WILL NEVER FAIL YOU."

FRANK LLOYD WRIGHT

If plants or materials that we touch and feel could talk to us, what would they be telling us about themselves?

I believe they are already talking to us because, if they are not, then how can we receive the vibrations from their presence, which influences our emotions and our state of mind?

What triggers those emotions when some things feel good or lead to a sensation of well-being, while others lead to sensations of anxiety and discomfort?

The goal is to help you become aware, so that you recognize the unique qualities that you can attune and sharpen your senses to. Although it has been discovered that human beings are perceptively inclined towards a range of warm colours and tones, every single one of us is a unique individual; we have slightly different range of colours and the specifics of our preferences is an exciting journey that we can discover for ourselves. I challenge you to become aware of materials and their unique relationships according to your personal interpretation of design.

BIOPHILIA

Humans are drawn to and fascinated by the natural world. We are driven by the desire to connect with other living beings, whether plants or animals. This is "biophilia": the innate tendency we all possess to connect with life and things vital, or the "love of life" in general.[29] We need to have more knowledge about the natural world, in particular the nuances and secret recipes that are embedded in it.

When you develop this sense, you will acquire an insatiable desire to improve your immediate living space or your workplace.

We shall now start to talk about biophilic design and unlock some of the reasons why it matters to our everyday life. Biophilia, according to the Oxford Dictionary, is the innate and genetically determined affinity human beings have with the natural world.[30] This exists in many different ways. It may be in the form of the physical properties of materials that exist in nature, or it may be in the way that we visually perceive (knowingly or unknowingly at times) the geometries and shapes existing in nature to follow certain principles and logic.

SIGNATURE OF MY ARCHITECTURE

Among the many buildings I have designed, the most memorable ones are those that integrate natural elements. Together with a vernacular attitude to design, I feel the best architecture stems from appropriating and reflecting what is around, to help our hearts and minds attain a very comfortable and quiet pleasure.

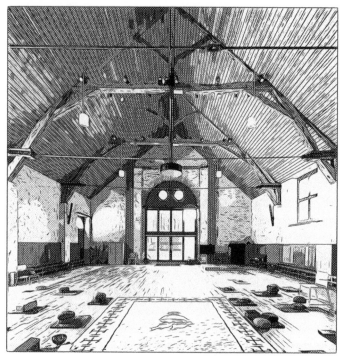

PHOTO: MEDITATION HALL OF THE WCCM BONNEAVAUX
MEDITATION CENTRE, POITIER, FRANCE.

Source: Author's own collection

One example is the Bonneavaux Meditation
Centre,[31] which was a project I was blessed
to have been involved in. It involved the con-
version of a 12th Century monastery into a
world-class meditation retreat centre, and it
illustrates vividly the principle of marrying
nature with the built space. The meditation
hall in that project is a space that connects

vibrationally very deeply with me when I stand in there and close my eyes.

This hall is perhaps one of the few pieces of completed design work that truly vibrates and connects to us through all six senses. I have included here a photograph to show how basic it is, but please don't be fooled. If I can use actual spaces to give definitions to words, this piece of work spells "sophisticated simplicity." It is a little unfair to try to describe it using words, and I suggest anyone who wishes to experience this to visit the place itself in Bonneavaux, Poitier, central France.

In a healthcare facility located in Carrickmines, Ireland, our design team was privileged to produce spaces that exude calm and portray an atmosphere of home and tranquillity. I include here a photo of an extremely simple waiting space. Complementing the natural light through the external façade, we incorporated a rather large print that reflects the natural outdoors. The subtle choices of matching colours and fabrics, along with the balanced use of wood as a base material, allows the heart rate to slow down and the mind to subconsciously relax.

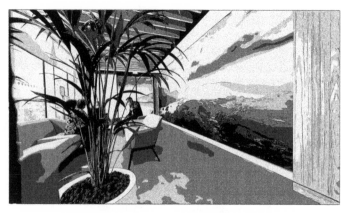

PHOTO: WELL-BEING CONSIDERED WAITING AREA IN THE
CARRICKMINES HEALTHCARE FACILITY, DUBLIN.

Source: Author's own collection

It houses research laboratories and integrates advanced design elements with the purest abstract elements from Mother Nature. An elevated landscaped walkway which I coined the "green ribbon" metaphorically and physically links the two towers of research lab spaces. The daylight-reflecting glass screens juxtaposed with the lush tropical green walls, topped by trellises which support creepers at the upper part of this exposed space, are intended to form what we call a "green carpet of shade."

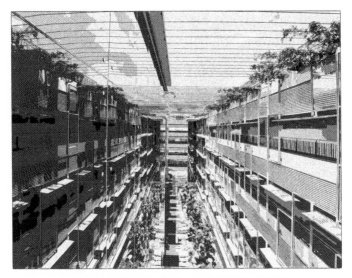

PHOTO: CENTRAL OPEN-TO-AIR ATRIUM ZONE WITH
GROWING CARPET OF CREEPERS AT CANOPY LEVEL.
CLEANTECH ONE, SINGAPORE.

Source: Author's own collection

The external façade of CTO is covered with a
configuration of carefully organised perforated
sheets. Each sheet that shields the corridors
from rain is punctuated with a range of circular holes, organised in a seemingly haphazard
way. The pattern on the sheets interacts with
the viewer's eyes depending on their distance
from the building. When the viewer is closer to
the building, the circular holes serve as small
viewing apertures. There is visual connection
with the outside, and the gentle breezes drawn
through the building's sides enters through

these punctured holes to improve the natural ventilation through the building. The magic happens when viewing the building from a distance. The building transforms into a soft-edged cube; some call it the "Japanese water-melon." This is because of an optical illusion created by the pattern of perforations forming a biophilic texture. And, to let you in on a secret, the pattern is based on photographs of trees I captured when I conceived the entire idea.

The abstraction and integration of nature's elements, including its flora and fauna, its geometric codes, its patterns and accents, etc., is biophilia.

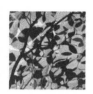  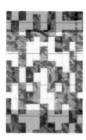 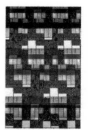

IMAGE: SERIES OF GRAPHICAL ADAPTIONS,
FROM PHOTO TO PERFORATION PATTERN.

It does not do justice to these projects to describe them in a few mere paragraphs here. I only wanted to reveal how biophilia and the integration of nature and its elements is a technique that can be deployed effectively by drawing on references from nature's shapes and geometries. When implemented with good balance, a space can exude a sense of calmness and serenity, simply by embedding this magical ingredient existing in abundance all around us.

THE NATURAL FLOW OF DESIGN IN MY OWN HOME

If we look at the types of materials that we can touch in our own homes, we will be able to identify that they fall broadly into certain groups. On the one hand, there are design elements that are directly extracted from nature like wood, clay and sand. On the other hand, there are more advanced materials that are manifested through more recent technological advances. These include steel, processed metals, and glass.

In my own home, I have selected and deliberately used a curated palette of wood together with naturally formed colours such as brass, bronze, and darker shades of grey. The type of wood that I particularly like to experiment with is birch ply, and I use birch ply in a multitude of ways in many of my design pieces. The natural patterns visible in birch ply are subtle but demonstrate the patterns of nature, while its lighter warm tone is a calming hue when used with other complementary materials and colours like brass and a grey that is almost black.

The way we mix and match materials can bring out the unique character of our home, the same way we express ourselves through the way we dress.

We see the world in colours. Even bright white light is a composite of the colour spectrum. Think of the rainbow! Colours, when put together, communicate to us in a way that can be pleasing or uncomfortable. The way that colours work is fundamentally informed by how nature processes its colour wavelengths. If we look at nature and the different shades of greens, blues, and browns and echo these colours in our own designs and our environments, there is a good chance that a degree of harmony can be created.

Although there are some standard approaches to how we interpolate and play with colours, each of us has different tastes, and these are informed by our cultural backgrounds and the way that we have been introduced to the appreciation of nature.

One of the challenges I put to you through this book is to identify the broad categories of materials and colours you surround yourself with, or are drawn to. Contrary to the belief that there is good design and bad design, I

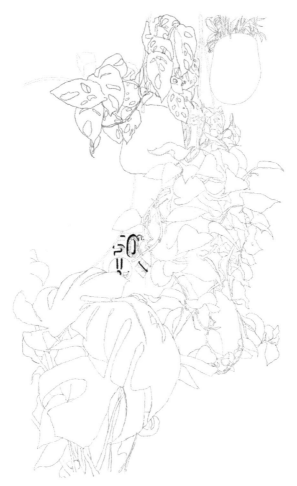

**DRAWING: LINE DRAWING OF INDOOR PLANTS IN MY
LIVING ROOM, BY IRIS AND I.**

prefer to believe that there is design that is true to you, and there is design that is foreign and not so identifiable to your culture.

Here you see a line drawing of indoor plants captured as lines on paper. It is a drawing jointly produced by my daughter Iris and I. As far as I am concerned, having plants in my home positively impacts me every day, and this extends beyond their sheer existence. Here they became the source material for this collaboration. The experience of creating this with my daughter embedded deep, pleasurable memories for me.

Through the act of drawing, placing lines onto paper, we are also firing up our senses of observation, perception and imagination. These are expressed through the way we coordinate our fingers and our hands, as controlled by our brains while we are seeing and thinking about shapes and objects. Much like journaling, which is the putting down of words relating to ideas and concepts we have in our brains, drawing has a similar power and effect. I prefer drawing and sketching to writing, as I believe they give us more back in return.

When creating a new space for my daughters, I identified two interconnected rooms for them, and this is a sketch by my younger daughter, Iris, when she was fascinated with how the space could be used.

This sketch shows how my younger daughter, Iris, conceived the possibility of an elevated bed, maximizing the space by also placing a study area below. There were various other details that she had in mind which were not included in the sketch, but I believe the sketch, together with the photograph next to it, shows the pure and naive ambition of a five-year-old's vision of how best to enhance their well-being in their own space.

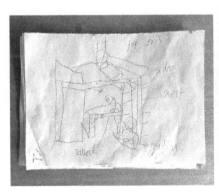 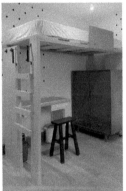

DRAWING: IRIS' SKETCH OF HER SPECIAL BUNK BED
AND THE EVENTUALLY CONSTRUCTED RESULT.

The inclusion of this sketch in this book is not to illustrate Iris's drawing capability. It is to demonstrate that a piece of drawing is a record or a manifestation of ideas in our mind. And it is not necessary for a drawing to be appreciated only when it subscribes to the stereotypical definition of art. (Side reminder: In some ways, the older and more informed we get, the more de-sensitised we become to them wonders of pure ingenuity because our yardstick has become fixated with conventional definitions.)

Here also, are some sketches for my elder daughter Ella's bespoke elevated bed, that I designed and created for our home. The processing of thoughts and ideas to create a design (in this case, a piece of furniture) is a journey of inception of concepts, modification, and creative problem-solving. I feel that designing is a productive endeavour that uses the right approach to seeing things around us. When we pay attention to what is around us, only then can we start to recognize what we might not have paid attention to before and build on it.

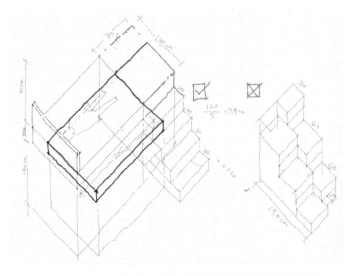

DRAWING: SKETCHES USED FOR DISCUSSION WITH MY DAUGHTER
FOR HER IMPROVISED BESPOKE RAISED BED.

BE OPEN TO YOUR
UNIQUE TASTES

Sharing how my personal spaces were con-
jured up and co-created with my daughters
is intended to inspire you to invest time with
your family and closest ones to do the same.
For this to work, you must embrace the methodology and the spirit of experimentation.
This is particularly true for grownups, whose
spirit of experimentation might have been
lost and needs to be relearned. We should

remember, however, that human beings have the privilege of being intuitively ambidextrous and have the skills to draw. Drawing is not a skill or talent only possessed by fine artists to display for a selected view. Each of us sees pictures in our brains and each of us remembers things via pictures rather than words.

The spirit here is to never remain with the status quo. We should always be in the process of learning, in whatever small way. By not experimenting and not taking chances, we are standing still and are not allowing ourselves to move forward. In the mindset of positive thinking and learning and growing, I believe that we are much better off if we move forward and arrive at the wrong place than if we do not journey at all. Experiment within your home and get a feel of the colours or designs that add a sense of joy to your being.

There are specific palettes of materials, colours, styles and, indeed, design genres that we can see online or in physical print magazines. We can use these to get impressions and form opinions of what we like and what we don't. In my view, it is irrelevant to use such sources as reference points of what is "right" or "wrong," design-wise. In fact, this process of inquiry is essentially a search for our own individuality, identifying our individual triggers for comfort, well-being and a sense of calm.

TRY THIS OUT

I would like to invite you to choose one space, just one, that is important to you in your own home, whether it is the bedroom, living space or dining area. Document this space in photographs, using your phone. Then write down some simple notes on those pictures about the type of materiality that exists in this particular space. Are the floor or wall surfaces made of wood, or plaster, or cement? Are there textiles such as fabric and carpet? Do you have plants indoors?

Organise the information you're writing down and consider whether what you've written about the palette you see in this space can be reduced to fewer, simpler words. Take five to ten minutes to think through whether there is any order to or priority of your senses that respond to these observations. Which of your senses was activated first? For example was it smell then sight? What do you feel? Be observant of how the room affects you. Are you calmer, or more active when you enter this space? Whether it is your workspace or a space to rest, notice what changes you feel to your well-being when you make a small change to the space.

This exercise should give you the inspiration to start to curate the materials in your space into a more organized and concise palette, one that is specific to your taste and your preferences, bespoke and individual. This leads me to an important question: What is the true and exact purpose of spaces in our homes and the workplace? Are you beginning to understand the deeper role they each have in your quest to become more well and to be happier every present moment?

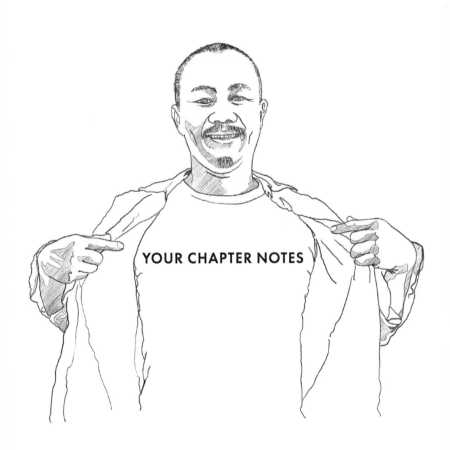
YOUR CHAPTER NOTES

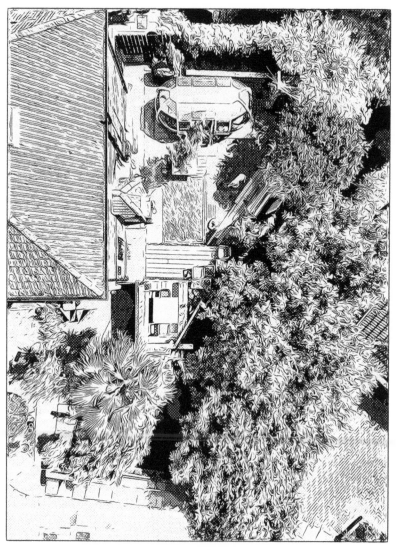

PHOTO: AERIAL VIEW OF THE GARDEN OF MY HOME.

CHAPTER 6

UNDERSTANDING THE FUNCTIONS OF SPACES

*"EVEN A COMMON, ORDINARY BRICK ...
WANTS TO BE SOMETHING MORE THAN IT IS.
IT WANTS TO BE SOMETHING BETTER THAN IT IS."*

LOUIS KAHN

We shape our spaces and our spaces, in turn, shape us.

We should actively invest our energy and attention into designing the environment around us. If we don't, we miss out on the benefit of these spaces helping us function better and more effectively. A simple way of explaining this is by considering your desk at work. Until you clear off your work desk and make it tidy, you simply cannot experience the impact this tiny footprint of less than half a square meter has on your ability to think and focus at your best.

Spaces where we dwell and operate every day – including where you are sitting right now as you read this – are not random spots where you happen to exist. Each space can allow you to be your best self, performing at your optimum. An operating theatre should not be just a space that happens to have some medical machinery and a large hanging spotlight above a metallic bed on wheels.

A place that is a bit of everything, in my view, becomes nothing. This is aligned with the broad objectives and principles of self-care. Just as when we try to multitask and perform many roles we do not achieve optimally, a space that has too many roles does not work in our favour. The moment certain qualities in a space become too fragmented the space loses its original intended use, so much so that it doesn't perform any purpose at all. When spaces perform and function too flexibly, meaning they do not have a dedicated purpose, they don't function effectively anymore.

For example, if we agree that the bedroom is a place to recharge, a place to recuperate and be our most intimate and innermost person, it must be that. It has to be just a place of rest, or it will exist in many different forms and try to work in a myriad of roles. We need to recognize that each space within the home or work environment has a fairly narrow set of purposes. There are key needs for some of these key spaces, and this awareness will trigger your thoughts to evaluate how each of the spaces surrounding you influence your day.

Studies have suggested that the use of the dining table as a space for office work during the pandemic was linked to an increase in burnout. Our minds use spatial cues to associate activities to the spaces that we use and interact with, and working from home has introduced to us a new challenge: the demarcation of work and personal boundaries.[32] At the onset of the global COVID-19 pandemic lockdown, it was not possible to have prepared in advance for the sudden implementation of working from home, and many people did not have the opportunity to consider the best way for them to function while doing so. Many experiments have been tried and lessons learned as a consequence, and I have been involved in projects to design bespoke solutions for working-from-home spaces that do not necessitate the use of spaces dedicated to other purposes, such as the dining room or the bedroom. This separation of spatial functions is important for both physical and mental well-being.[33]

Such observations can stimulate your personal insights to come up with ideas about how each space can work better for you personally.

You will be able to exercise a greater sense of presence during each of your daily activities and routines. In particular, you will be able to achieve quality time with yourself and your loved ones.

YOUR BEDROOM

Almost all architects and spatial designers are taught that in modernism there is one basic rule: form follows function. In simple terms, this stipulates that the shape and physical properties of a building or space are to allow effective inhabitation, as well as to facilitate the way that that space is prescribed to be used.

The second principle is less is more, which relates to reducing unnecessary visual clutter of materials, design qualities, and information. Such clutter happens if one is not focused on the true essence of the space.

I adhere to these two principles, but probably in a more adjusted and appropriate way.

Let's talk about sleeping, for example. Sleeping is one of a human being's vital daily activities. We each spend around one-third of our entire lifetimes asleep, and the function of sleep is for the body to readjust, recalibrate, recuperate, and to be ready for the non-sleep two-thirds.[34]

Obviously, sleeping is an important activity for the human body and brain. And in modern times, we do this in the sanctuary of our bedroom. During our cave-dwelling times, sleep would have occurred in a part of the cave where the family unit slept and restored energy. This part of the cave would have to be well protected to prevent unpegged danger or threats.

Have you ever considered whether your bedroom is working for you? Does it make you feel safe and secure, and does it exude serenity? Does your bedroom serve its purpose of letting you be yourself while also recharging you for the non-sleeping hours of your lifetime?

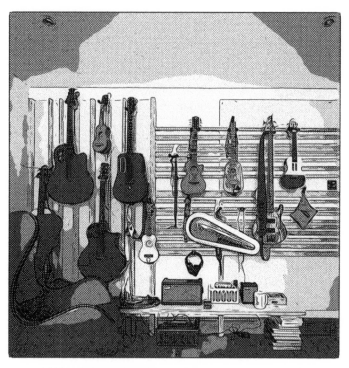

PHOTO: MUSIC LIFTS THE SOUL, AND BENEFITS MY WELL-BEING.
MY STRING INSTRUMENTS COLLECTION.

My own bedroom is my cave. The wall that
I see when I wake up is covered with a large
composition of three printed screens showing
the woodlands nearby, where I have spent
much time meditating and re-learning to be
myself. Lining another wall are all my musical instruments, a collection that I have built
up over recent years, on a functional hanging surface for this equipment I use regularly.

Metaphorically, the printed woodlands photo and the wall of ukuleles and guitars are no different to cave paintings I would have made if this was really my cave made of rock.

Because this is my personal space, it is also constructed with a warm tone of materiality: birch ply. Almost every single piece of furniture is designed and handcrafted by me: self-built items are more pleasurable to use, but also difficult to replace. So, the tone of well-being embedded in my design advocacy is also conscious of sustainability.

The wall with windows is installed with motorised blackout blinds. This has been one of the best investments, equipment-wise, in my home. It means that I can, at the press of a button, turn the space into one that is almost pitch dark, allowing me to be attuned to my natural circadian rhythms. Darkness welcomes melatonin, leading to sleep time, and light triggers cortisol's release so that we become fresh and ready in the mornings.

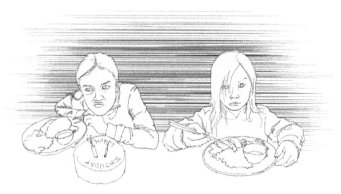

DRAWING: MY DAUGHTERS POSING FOR A MOCK UNHAPPY MEALTIME LOOK.

HAPPY MEAL

What, to you, is a happy meal? Is it about the food, the actual taking in of nutrition? Perhaps it is a sumptuous breakfast, a hearty fry-up, or something that is lean and part of a well-managed diet. Or, maybe, you will be thinking of McDonald's, but if we think of a meal that is happy, we are thinking about the environment or the ambience, the people we are with, together with the conversations and the interactions, the smiles, laughter, and perhaps even the arguments or the differences of opinion, the exchange of ideas and debates that we have over food.

Do you agree that good kitchens make happy meals? Do you believe that the quality of the design and the way that a space functions has a direct influence and impact on how we make and enjoy a meal? For me, the kitchen is the precursor to the dining table. The preparation of a meal, even the laying of the table, is akin to a ritual. Whenever possible, I love having all kinds of friends over for a meal, no matter how simple it is. I see making a meal as a celebration, a blessing of being able to dwell in moments of creating food. The flavours of what I make are seasoned with the conversations we have while making the meal. This means that I am a keen advocate for open kitchens, or at least those that have an opening that connects the kitchen to where the others might be: for example, sitting at a modified bar counter. In my view, the visual treat of being able to participate in the activity of preparing food is great entertainment. Pardon the pun, but I call this a feast for both the host as well as the guests.

DESIGNING YOUR MEMORIES

Is your dining room dedicated to the act of eating? In the modern lifestyle that we lead, the dining room is often associated with catching up on the news, spending time on social media and online shopping, and digital device time.

If we were to strip away these forms of distraction, we would understand that the dining room can serve us emotionally and physically. The interactions over a dining table lead to building memories, by physically connecting with, interacting and bonding with our family and friends.

Often, we do not pay attention to these attributes of the key spaces of our homes, and consequently, they become just transient moments of our everyday time. I think that, for us to have self-care and self-love, to be fully present, and to use every single moment when we breathe and we are alive, these seemingly transient spaces can indeed work for us in amazing ways.

I remember an acted-out experiment in The Social Dilemma, whereby a family was told how much of their mealtimes were being usurped by technology. As a way to try and highlight this point, the mother of the family bought a unique jar that had a time-based lock integrated into it. The family agreed that everyone would put their mobile phones into this jar for the next 30 or 45 minutes, during which the family was to spend time together to eat their family meal. Even though all of the devices were set to silent mode, they still vibrated. According to the experiment, the daughter was so uncomfortable that eventually, after having restrained herself for quite a while, she took the jar and smashed it, simply to be able to see which of her friends was messaging her, either on social media or directly.

This is an illustration of how powerful the psychology of user experience and user interface design is in our technology and gadgets. There is a great deal of insight and thoughtful expertise placed into the designing of the vibrations, the ring tones or the graphics of the little icons that we receive. These carefully assessed and intelligently designed interfaces and details are intended to compel us to react. In fact, they trigger the reptilian brain, the part of our brain that is a direct impulse without rational processing or evaluating, to instinctively respond.

Being aware of this can give us back a lot of power. It can give us the opportunity to deliberately reduce the way that such details can influence our mind space. It gives us the chance to recalibrate and make decisions to control how much attention and mind space and time we give to a device.

A personal story I want to share is one that is deep in my memory. I spent very little time with my grandfather, but I occasionally had breakfast with him. Being a migrant to Singapore from China, he had worked as a labourer and had gone through very tough times, so he was frugal. His typical breakfast at the coffee shop would involve a half-boiled egg, maybe a slice of toast and a cup of coffee. I remember vividly the way that he would break the half-boiled egg into the saucer that comes with the coffee cup. He would slurp down the half-boiled egg together with some pepper and soy sauce and follow it by pouring into the same saucer the coffee to wash down the egg. I was told that he did this because of how precious the protein from the egg was. He would make sure not to waste any of the egg and ate every little bit of it that was left on the saucer.

I mention this memory to illustrate how the time spent over a meal is, to a degree, very little about the actual consumption of the food, and more about the emotional story and the experience of being together at the dining table. Some of these memories that might not be extremely significant as events are embedded very deep in our memory banks. In the moments when we are quiet and reflect, we can recall some of these events which are significantly inscribed as part of our childhoods.

This is why I encourage anyone reading this book to enjoy being present in every space and time. Be present at this very moment, in whatever you are doing.

The Chinese word for "present" is 礼物. This refers to the alternative meaning of the word "present" as a "gift." Borrowing this idea, you can see that by being present, you are dedicating a present to your future self. This is a neat idea to encourage ourselves to be fully present.

For the spaces around us to work better, we have to learn how to curate the functions within these spaces. The ability to curate must be learned along a personal journey; it is not a taught exercise. The stories I share about my own personal spaces are intended to communicate the methodologies I have tested out, for you to supercharge your own learning and experimental process.

We need to understand that space is just a medium or a conduit to achieving certain root functions or purposes. Each space should also serve the objective of uplifting and enhancing, holistically, our states of well-being. By simplifying the spaces around us and dedicating certain spaces to serve only a selected range of functions, we are helping ourselves to form productive habits.

One example could be the way that we might store the cookie jar on the top shelf of a cupboard. Keeping it in a slightly more remote part of the kitchen is important to someone who is trying to abstain or trying to cut down on the consumption of biscuits and sweet things. It is counterintuitive to have the cookie jar nearby if you're trying to not eat cookies, and it is more conducive to those efforts to store the cookie jar where it requires more effort to access. Experiments and analysis have demonstrated that this is far more effective than just allowing yourself to have easy access to them.

Designing spaces, and making them work better for us, is simple. How we can focus the moments that we have to be more productive, at any single point in time, relies on our ability to be in a state of well-being.

As a reminder, we are never in stasis, and in every single moment of our living day, there are opportunities for us to observe how we might improve our present day, as well as the following. By making these decisions and making the small tweaks, we move forward in the tiniest way. It's a small but big adjustment, and it gets us closer to our spaces functioning in a way that suits our lifestyles better.

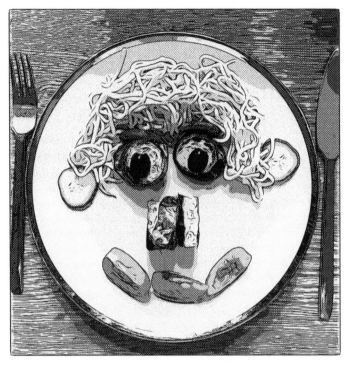

PHOTO: HAPPY MEALS TO CELEBRATE AND INJECT HAPPY INGREDIENTS INTO THE MAKING OF MEALS FOR THE FAMILY CHILDREN.

Source: Author's own collection

TRY THIS OUT

Having discussed the three spaces in your
home that serve key purposes, I challenge you
to create more impact in your own spaces.

Choose one space that is important to you,
preferably at home. It could be, for example,
your bedroom, the living space or the dining
area. Journal the three most important reasons why such a space that you have chosen is
special and relevant to you.

UP NEXT ...

There is so much to connect who we are today
with our ancestors. As far as I am concerned,
I believe we are still fundamentally cavemen.

In the next chapter I will share some further
insights and connections on how our spaces
play an intrinsic role in our mental state of
well-being and happiness.

YOUR CHAPTER NOTES

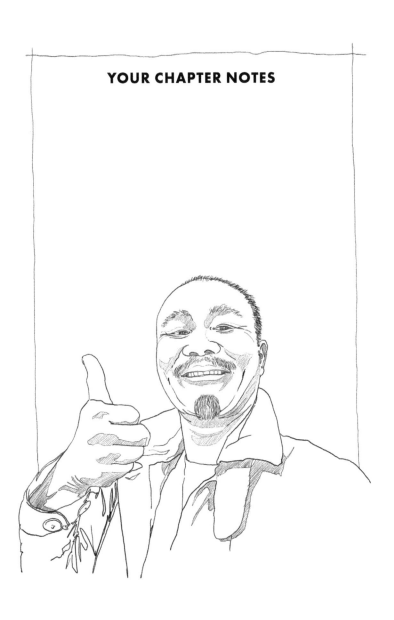

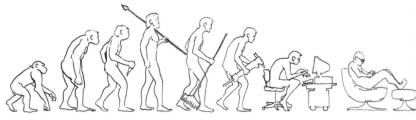

DRAWING: EVOLUTIONARY POSES OF THE CAVEMEN,
PRESCRIBED BY HIS DAILY ROUTINES.

Source: Authors own drawing

CHAPTER 7

MODERN DAY CAVEMEN

"YOU CAN TAKE THE PERSON OUT OF THE STONE AGE, NOT THE STONE AGE OUT OF THE PERSON."[35]

NIGEL NICHOLSON

The caveman is a descriptive word that literally means men who live in caves. The cave of primitive man has evolved to become our homes, ones that are built. And we have today an wide array of interventions and treatments we can apply to our modern caves. Do we still adorn the walls with our markings to record our hunting trips or the unusual flora and fauna we have encountered? Instead of ferns and moss naturally finding a foothold, are there indoor plants?

For me, I strongly believe that we are a modern and slightly more technologically advanced version of cavemen. Almost all of our intuitive mindset and spatial registers are still active, and function in our current environment.

Although we are a lot more advanced and do things in a more sophisticated way, we are hardwired to still operate like cavemen. I often jokingly remark that we can indeed be hardwired to refer to the steel and glass constructions of modern cities, but that will be in another hundred thousand years' time. After all, that is how much time has lapsed to lead to our brains being calibrated the way they are today.

When I design and set up my home office space, I like to sit where I can look out to a distant view, and also have my back facing my bookshelves or walls that have no doors or openings. Psychologically, I prefer to have anyone or anything that can approach me within my line of sight. This is akin to the settings of good fortune in some feng shui teachings, like positioning oneself on elevated ground to be able to look out to sea, which means you can have first sightings of any enemies as well as the incoming harvest from the seas. I think this is us thinking as cavemen.

If we cannot go back in time to change how our perception and modus operandi have evolved, the next best thing is to understand it as best as we can and conduct today's tasks with them in mind.

INSTINCTUAL NEEDS

Despite how different we might look, we are no more than iterative versions of the same cavemen. Alongside our evolution, the desire for overall knowledge growth and the acquiring of new skills is part of the ambition to seek happiness. Our instinct for happiness derives primarily from our cavemen times.

In every species of living creature, including in humans, the brain is primarily driven by the need to prevent the demise of the species, through ensuring survival and procreation. Because of the need to stay alive, we as a tribe also have a deep desire to be connected, to belong to a group, and to be appreciated and liked. The need to become an appreciated member of a larger group allows our continued existence and protection against enemies or predators. Anthropologists believe that other homo-species disappeared because of their inability to cluster adequately to battle against threats and predators. In a way, ganging up was at one point a necessary course of action that eventually became second nature.

This logic is one of the key pillars the designers and creators of social media embedded into the original algorithm. In the documentary "Social Dilemma,"[36] a group of early-generation social media platform creators and academic researchers articulated how their work involved an exceptionally complex understanding of the human being's psychological needs and cravings. The original goal of social media was to be raise the connectedness of human being through the internet, to bring about a great sense of belonging. Ironically, this algorithm is today causing us much stress and discomfort, due to the resultant business model to aggressively market in order to expand and prolong every individual's screen time. This awareness of how a positive motivation has been transformed is the basis of my exploration of how the narrative can be changed.

I believe we must first start to understand our instinctual tendencies: that part of ourselves that automatically directs us towards feeling good. This is the same sensation that the original beta versions of social media were aiming to achieve.

Feeling good is the most basic step of our quest for happiness. While some current research suggests that our instinct is aligned with the objective of avoiding unhappiness, my personal belief is that this attitude is too passive. If you understand the stories I have shared in my life's twists and turns, you should be able to recognise me as one who takes action toward what I want and believe in, not to avoid discomfort.

EGM[37]

Even as cavemen our brains were already intuitively organized to seek happiness. This search for happiness can be understood under the heading of EGM. I use EGM as an acronym to help us remember, just as it represents the words in the business arena, Extraordinary General Meeting. An EGM in business is a meeting we call when we have a special agenda, a special important issue to deal with which cannot wait for the routine annual general meeting.

E stands for Experiences, **G** for growth and learning, and **M** for meaning and purpose. While there are many ways to understand happiness, I have found that this approach is the easiest to interpret and the easiest to enter into the discourse and the study of happiness.

E STANDS FOR EXPERIENCES

When we say **experiences**, we refer to the moments when we have a positive emotion and a positive reflection on any moment in time. These experiences can be through either the things we do, or the objects that we possess or acquire.

The reason why many queue up, perhaps even overnight, in anticipation of being among the first to own the latest iPhone model, is because of the thrill and exhilaration we experience when we obtain a brand-new product that we believe is going to transform something in our daily lives. I did not queue up for the new iPhone, but I certainly beamed with joy for half a day when I acquired the latest edition. Justifying to myself that I now have more features that I need, I was truly happy. Or, at the very least, I was experiencing a good dose of materialistic bliss.

Experiences can also be positive doses of happiness from a holiday, a shared moment with your loved ones such as a candlelight dinner, a romantic excursion, or a family outing. One of the properties of experiences is that they are time-based. These experiences, regardless of how intensive or how moderated they are or how deliberate, how intentional or how by chance they happen to occur, exist for a limited period of time.

Sometimes a positive response might last as short as 90 seconds. In the case of memories from major holidays, these feelings might last as long as weeks and perhaps even months. Nevertheless, after a certain point in time, the feeling from the experience dwindles and fades.

G STANDS FOR GROWTH
AND LEARNING

Growth and Learning are basic instincts of a human being. These instincts attach themselves to the need for survival.

By the end of 2020, after I was able to stabilise my mental imbalance with medication, I realised how much I had robbed myself of Growth and Learning. In the previous ten years, I had read one book; in the following twelve months, I read 23. And even though I might only have absorbed about 10-20 per cent of the potential learnings contained within them, that is far more than the ten years before. I was happy learning. I might not be becoming wiser, but I was happy because, to me, I felt that I was. It was like magic.

In order for human beings to survive, we have to continuously be creative, innovate and acquire new skills. Think of the cavemen who discovered and realized that sparks caused by heat and friction when combined with air and kindling can create flames.

In my mind, I visualize a particular scene in the movie "Cast Away"[38] with Tom Hanks, when his character is stranded on an island. Alone and stripped to basics, he had to survive on the rudimentary instincts of a hunter gatherer, so he was living on coconut water. When he found a way to start a fire, that particular scene, which lasted almost two minutes or so, showed the exhilaration we feel when we have discovered something so crucial and important that is a primary element necessary for survival.

Growth and learning in our modern day can be illustrated by more contemporary examples, such as when one learns another language, or when one takes up dance lessons. Growth and learning may be in the form of knowledge or it might be in the form of physical skills. For the longest time, growth and learning has been one of the intrinsic ways our brains derive and attain pleasure and satisfaction.

But what has happened to growth and learning today? The problem that we have is that we have created a mindset that growth and learning is for children and not so much for adults. If you are a parent, remember the moment when your infant, probably at the age of between 10 and 15 months and after a prolonged period of trying to stand with support, took their first steps. The pure joy and delight and the satisfaction and sense of accomplishment that you saw on the child's face is the exact visual illustration of happiness through growth and learning.

Sadly, the education systems that we adults have created have gradually and in a very disciplined and organized way instilled into our minds that learning is something that is not a happy thing to do. This has come about by the methodology of learning requiring tests, exams and other triggers of high anxiety. If we can deal with this, we can bring back growth and learning to serve its pure purpose of generating pleasure and happiness.

M STANDS FOR MEANING AND PURPOSE

For us to exist, it is not enough to have positive experiences combined with awareness and the acquisition of new skills and growth. In our minds, we are also perpetually wondering why we exist, that each of us must be here because of a bigger logic that we fit into, like a giant jig-saw puzzle. Here in the category of meaning and purpose, we are dealing with how each individual exists as part of a group, or a piece of a larger jigsaw puzzle.

When you change your baby's nappy, it should be one of the most unpleasant experiences you will ever have, because of the human waste that your fingers will be touching, and that you will be seeing and smelling. However, I'm sure that most parents will remember this as a time when you had a lot of fun, laughing and playing and making jokes with your young infant who didn't even understand, but who reciprocated with smiles and giggles.

I share this image based on visual recollections of me with my first born, Ella. She was so little and laid out in the shallow Corian washbasin of our Singapore home at the time. I changed her nappy so many times I was adept at the operation, without any need to even be aware of what I was doing. Instead, what I was doing was experiencing the pure joy, and deep happiness of bonding with my most precious one. It is bewildering how an act that is so uncomfortable, if not disgusting, involving our hands handling the human waste of another, can actually be pleasant. But yet those of us who have children can relate to it. Something more sophisticated and unknown to our logical processing must be happening.

At a neurological level, our brain releases tiny chemical messengers called neuropeptides to help fight off stress, alongside other neurotransmitters like dopamine, serotonin and endorphins. This is because we are at that very moment having a very special experience of our human existence based on the logic that we exist to serve and to be part of other beings' lives. I believe that the cavemen (mother or father) also felt a sense of pride and comfort that there was a successor to the tribal existence.

Other ways meaning and purpose can be understood is when we serve as a member of our community, as part of a charity group or a religious organization or a sporting or social club. When we exist as a member of a collective that has similar beliefs, does certain activities or shares an opinion on certain subjects, we understand and psychologically have an awareness of our joy and happiness through meaning and purpose.

For us to experience EG and M or to understand and practice EG and M in today's world, we have to perhaps reinterpret how our caveman brain can be adjusted based on today's technology and lifestyle and everyday routines.

FOREST IN OUR MODERN CAVES

Let me draw an image in your mind. Imagine yourself as a caveman. When you as caveman look out towards the horizon and to the space beyond the cave, you would typically see forests and foliage, bushes, trees, perhaps a stream and, basically, natural surroundings.

Imagine that one of the bushes moves suddenly. Your instinctive response will be to immediately shift your attention and focus on that particular spot. Why? This is because there are two likely reasons why the bush suddenly moved. It will be either that at the spot lies the next meal, or that it conceals a sabre-toothed tiger, ready to pounce and enjoy you as its next meal.

This particular way our brains work, and the intuitive response by the limbic section of our brain moving the eyes to pay attention to the possible threat, is spontaneous. This is one example of, and an illustration that there are indeed many aspects of our brain's workings that are hardwired from caveman times.

This illustration is also used to bring attention to the way that we might curate our spaces so that there is no visual distraction, in order for the brain to focus on and be more productive in doing what we need to do. If there is something in the background that doesn't belong, it can cause distraction, even if it is in our peripheral vision.

For this understanding to develop into something useful to you every day, I recommend you put in a little bit of effort in designing your own home to begin to discover your comfort zones. The comfort zone is akin to when you have lived far away from your family home and you come back to your mother's cooking. Regardless of what your mom's cooking is like and whether it is technically of a high standard, you will appreciate your mom's cooking because your mom's cooking is like coming home.

I recommend everyone get connected with their gut instinct. There is no equipment necessary. Just use your gut instinct, close your eyes, and listen to your body's response to certain details. The awareness of how to hack your mind to motivate yourself to work in your own favour is a very special skill requiring practice.

In a world filled with modern technology, it is important to recognize the basic rules of what affects us to our innermost cores. Our instinct to remain alive and to survive as a species require us to form tribes and gang up to defend territories and protect our young. There is also the core evolutionary nature to reproduce and sustain a species through reproduction.

These are essential aspects to understand and appreciate, and they overlap with our understanding of the functional notions of the spaces that we dwell and operate in today.

TRY THIS OUT

Identify three objects that you instinctively find comfortable to hold in your hands. Your choice can be based on the sense of touch, the items colours or its materiality. This might be your mobile phone, your watch, a piece of jewellery, furniture or an ornament.

Study and journal about the physical attributes of those objects. Are they sharp? Do they have curved edges? Do they fit into your palm? Do the objects suggest natural shapes or profiles or other aspects that make you comfortable? This exercise will help to hone your eye to decipher and appreciate the likeness between more desirable and pleasurable details, which for you register safety, comfort, and positive memories.

UP NEXT ...

The next thing we are going to talk about is how, as homo sapiens, we are social creatures who band together to survive and procreate. This will then link directly with the impact of the physical environment, the way its architecture and design properties produce either conducive or negative effects on the way the spaces can function.

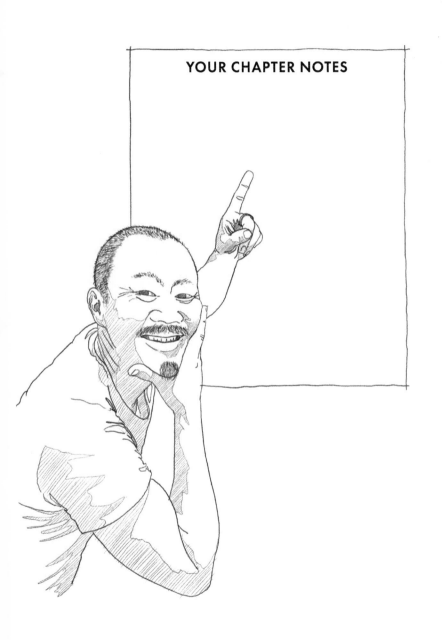

YOUR CHAPTER NOTES

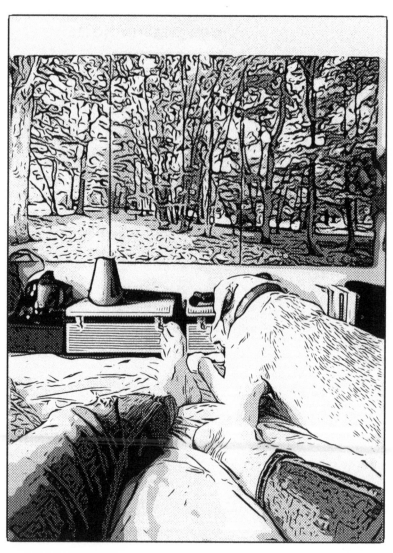

PHOTO: WHAT I SEE FROM MY BED IN MY BEDROOM.

CHAPTER 8

TRIBES:

We Love Being
Part of a Gang

*"HUMAN BEINGS CAN'T HELP IT: WE NEED TO
BELONG. ONE OF THE MOST POWERFUL OF OUR
SURVIVAL MECHANISMS IS TO BE PART OF A TRIBE,
TO CONTRIBUTE TO (AND TAKE FROM) A GROUP
OF LIKE-MINDED PEOPLE. WE ARE DRAWN TO
LEADERS AND TO THEIR IDEAS."*[39]

SETH GODIN

The first thing many of us do when we
wake up in the morning is look at ourselves
in the mirror. I am curious to know, where
is your mirror? Is it in your bedroom or in
your bathroom? Have you ever asked yourself the purpose of a mirror? Besides dress-
ing and personal grooming, how else can a
mirror serve you?

Focusing on how we see ourselves is a method
of self-care that is beginning to be pushed
to the lowest ranks of priorities in our busy

schedules. This is not to say that we need to attain self-adoration, but we need to have a high degree of self-respect and self-recognition for us to feel confident that we can move through our day and be effective. More and more, studies show that for our mental health, we need to work on ourselves first, to appreciate our own abilities and existence and relevance before we think about what we can do with and for others.

When I was working on my recovery from depression, I spent a long period routinely journaling and self-reflecting. There were days when I wrote and could not explain why my tears flowed uncontrollably. Finally, I reached the conclusion that my existence was to serve. It didn't matter to me whether I attained the type of success that our materialistic world considers to be fame or wealth: my goal was to live my every day to fulfil my meaning and purpose.

YOUR BEDROOM

To be comfortable requires an environment where we can experience a strong sense of safety and serenity. Which space do we turn our attention to first, if we accept that spaces matter? It is most natural to start with either where we spend the most time, or where the most important activity happens.

One space we should turn our attention to improving is our bedrooms. We need to ask ourselves what's holding us back from doing something for ourselves to make our ability to rest more effective.

I shared details of my bedroom in an earlier chapter, now it is time to go deeper into how yours can be. Each of us ought to have our bedroom space the way it can serve us best. It is important that we understand that this serves a wider purpose. It is not self-gratifying or self-indulgent, because for us to serve and be an effective part of a community, we have to care for ourselves first.

This instinctive need to care for ourselves will allow us to fulfil our desire to be part of a larger group, to be part of our tribe or tribes. Spaces that are carefully considered and improved are more effective places for us to bond, connect and collaborate.

Think about how often you reflect on your own personal spaces. Ask yourself whether they serve you or if they merely exist. Whenever you are at work, during the course of the day pay attention to the desk and work-space that surrounds you.

In the post-pandemic era, many of us worked from home for a lot of our endeavours and tasks. When you have piles of materials, documents, and papers stacked up right in front of you, have you ever asked whether that has any impact on you? Does it dampen your spirit and bring you down, reducing your ability to be effective and to focus?

One of the easy things that you can do for yourself as part of the self-care ritual is to declutter your desk and the space that surrounds you. It has been proven that the ability to see clarity in the physical environment translates to the ability to see clarity in your mind space. Our brain is so powerful that it is constantly searching for visual information to interpret; giving it too much is often a cause of our minds becoming overwhelmed.

THE SPACE FOR SELF

Self-care and self-love are two concepts that are often used interchangeably, but there are distinctive differences embodied within these two concepts. Self-care refers to the intentional actions taken to maintain or improve one's physical, emotional, and mental health. Self-love, on the other hand, refers to the positive regard and appreciation one has for oneself.

While self-care and self-love are related, it is possible to engage in one without the other. For example, someone may engage in self-care activities like exercising, eating well, and getting enough sleep, but they may not necessarily love themselves. On the other hand, someone may have a deep sense of self-love, but they may not prioritize their own physical or emotional needs.

Self-care is often a component of self-love, but self-love is not always a component of self-care. It can sometimes be motivated by a desire to improve oneself or meet societal expectations, or to fulfil the needs of others rather than oneself. In some instances, in fact quite often, I observe that self-care is carried out at the expense of self-love. Quite an irony.

Self-love involves developing a positive relationship with oneself, which includes treating yourself with kindness, respect, compassion, and empathy. In short, self-love is about accepting yourself as you are, flaws and all. It is more a state and attitude of the mind, and less about the actual actions or things that we pursue.

In summary, while self-care and self-love are related concepts, they do have distinct differences. Like we say, the devil is in the detail. It is possible to engage in one without the other, and both are important for holistic and overall well-being. The diagram of the two overlapping circles included here illustrates this understanding.

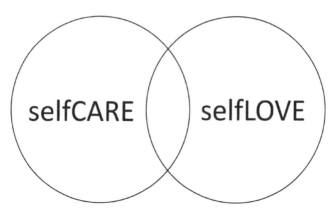

DIAGRAM: THE OVERLAPPING BUT ALSO SLIGHTLY DIFFERENT CONCEPTS OF SELFLOVE VERSUS SELFCARE.

We might start to wonder if there can be too much self-caring and self-loving. Interestingly, our ability to give ourselves some degree of care and love also affects how we are perceived by others.

WHAT IS THE DIFFERENCE BETWEEN
SELF-CARE AND SELF-LOVE?

Self-love is not about being infatuated with yourself. Recognizing that needing a place of solitude for ourselves is a basic component that we need in order to dwell and appreciate our own existence. This appreciation allows us to be fully present and for the cognitive mind to be able to process and advance further.

THE PERFUME CHARISMA
EXPERIMENT[40]

This was a study carried out which examined the effectiveness of one's own portrayal of confidence. It aimed to look at the way that our self-presentation of confidence affects the way we are perceived.

A group of male volunteers was invited to take part in the experiment. Each of them made a speech, introducing themselves and speaking about their likes, their dislikes, and anything else that might differentiate them as interesting individuals. None of the participants were informed of what the experiment was about because this might negate the actual findings. They were informed that their speech would be recorded and then shown to other participants who would then appraise it and respond directly to what they say.

Unbeknownst to them, some of them were randomly selected to be sprayed with perfume. This was done subtly so as not to influence them in any particular way. The recorded speeches were then shown to a group of observers, who would then rate how attractive they found each speaker and how persuasive and charismatic they found the speaker to be.

The study found that the speakers who were sprayed with perfume ranked highest in terms of attractiveness and persuasiveness. Those who were sprayed with perfume somehow understood subliminally that the perfume would make them more confident and more attractive, and actually presented themselves more confidently and more attractively.

The relevance of this story is to show that in exercising self-care, we can project that self-esteem to others. The way that we exercise care for ourselves directly affects our ability to be perceived positively and hence to be liked by and become an effective member of any community or tribe we would like to be part of. In other words, getting ourselves to be in a good state is the most important beginning of all forms of care. It has the added effect of increasing our (ability to fit) effectiveness of fitting into the tribe we identify with.

Any tribe that we belong to provides us with a sense of belonging. When we are in a space with others, we have a much higher chance of growing and flourishing and moving towards accomplishing our goals. Conversely, being alone means we lack the ability to calibrate, and we often end up focusing on issues that do not matter, leading to a lack of success which in turn draws us into the negative spiral of feeling bad about ourselves.

Tribes can exist in many different shapes and forms. They can be virtual and notional groupings of people with the same interests or agenda, or they might involve gatherings at actual venues. We can each also be a member of a variety of tribes.

In today's environment and the way that we work in society, it is not possible to stay isolated. It never has been possible, since the start of humanity, to be alone, to be a hermit, and to think that we can conquer it all by ourselves. Each of us needs to be a member of larger groups of various sizes. This serves both purposes of satisfying the need to belong in our minds, as well as being able to accomplish larger goals.

Commonalities become the glue that brings people together and this commonality is the very essence of a collective passion. Having a shared passion brings us the chance for a sense of achievement and an elevated state of mental well-being along the path of searching for happiness.

THE AUDITORY SENSE
OF BELONGING

One of the many tribes that I belong to involves music and playing the ukulele. Coming from a poor family, I didn't get an opportunity to learn a musical instrument during my childhood. Music lessons were not something within our means. I always told myself that I would, one day, be capable of playing some form of music.

About 15 years ago, I decided that there had to be a musical instrument that I could master, or at least that I could play even in the most basic way. Since I always liked string instruments, I fancied the guitar. However, the time I had to invest to practice on a six-stringed guitar was a little bit too much for my busy schedule. So I decided that I could manage four strings, the ukulele.

Being able to play several string instruments today has boosted my confidence and more than compensated for earlier times when I was a stranger to music. It not only gave me a sense of having exercised self-care and self-love, but it also connected me to tribes of ukulele groups and convinced me that I belong, and I enjoy belonging.

What gifts have you given yourself? This world offers so much in terms of sensory input, it is important to explore our own potential and to find new tribes. This is indeed part of self-care. Under one roof, in a space of support and love, we flourish and build our sense of self-esteem.

TRY THIS OUT

Journal to identify the aspects of your everyday life that you can sense an inner voice, an internal commitment to. Describe them as callings. Have you come across any instinctive preferences or desires to do certain things or to move in a certain direction?

This journaling exercise is to help you to understand and move towards a group or a community, a society or a tribe that you would like to belong to. To practice growth, join and motivate yourself to become a member of a tribe. The question here is, which tribe, which society, which group or collection of people with the same affinity to a subject will you belong to? For me it was music; for you, it could be art, or a sport.

On a related note, to help your self-reflection process, think about the space you can use at home to journal and develop this mental landscape of your motivation towards the tribe. Identify this spot as a regular space for your reflections. This helps to condition your brain to the association of this specific pocket of space with the activity of introspective me-time.

Additional tip to ponder:

Your home is your sanctuary, have you noticed what part of your home do you feel most relaxed? And what kind of surroundings are they?

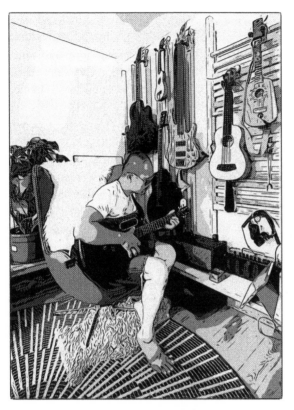

PHOTO: PART OF MY HOME DEDICATED FOR
MY MUSIC PRACTICE, WHICH ALSO SERVES AS
A GOOD SPOT FOR READING.

THE BOTTOM LINE

Identify three tribes that you belong to. One
of them will be, of course, your family unit.

But identify three other tribes that you belong to in addition to your family unit. Write down what attributes these groups have and which aspects of these you appreciate and which makes you continue to attend its activities. This might be a group of old classmates that you keep in touch with. Which spaces do you meet at and have the best time?

Spend at least five minutes writing, for each tribe, about the space that brings the most joy. Use the technique of closing your eyes and visualizing the space where the main activity of the tribe or group tends to be carried out.

Are there any specific parameters that enable the emotional senses of belonging, giving and serving, to be more enjoyable? From your perspective, what are they? Consider both the hardware, that is the space, and the software, the activities and the discussions, and how they matter.

UP NEXT ...

In the next chapter I will share with you three particular zones in your own home where you can, by yourself, implement tweaks and changes to make them serve you better. It is time to make some exciting changes!

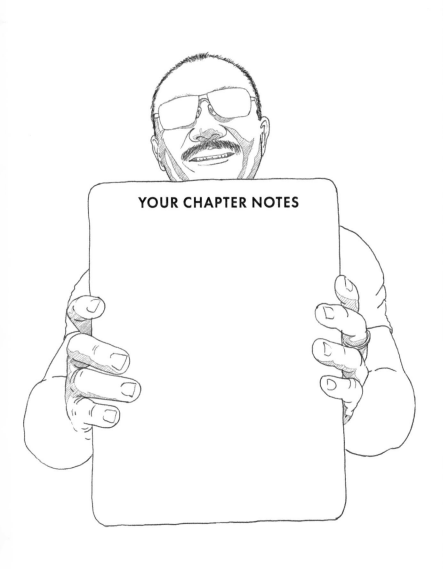

YOUR CHAPTER NOTES

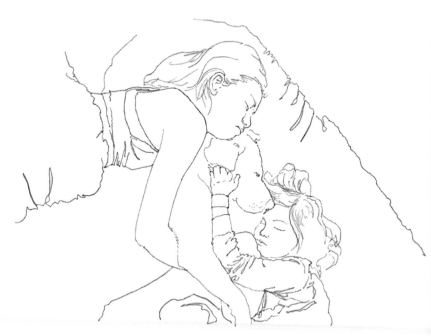

DRAWING: SLEEP TIME, FOR MY DAUGHTERS AND
ROXIE OUR LABRADOR RETRIEVER.

CHAPTER 9

DKZzzz (DINING/ KITCHEN/SLEEP):

The First Three Spaces in
Which to Start the Well-Being
and Happiness Hack at Home

*"ARCHITECTURE IS REALLY ABOUT WELL-BEING.
I THINK THAT PEOPLE WANT TO FEEL GOOD IN A
SPACE ... ON THE ONE HAND IT'S ABOUT SHELTER,
BUT IT'S ALSO ABOUT PLEASURE."*

ZAHA HADID

D stands for Diet, K for Kitchen, and Zzzz
represents sleep. These letters are extracted
from a parallel online teaching resource of
the WHAD movement.[41]

The areas in your home where you can achieve
the fastest results involve critical reflection
about what we do a lot, and where we do a lot
of these activities: namely, eating and sleeping.

It is not surprising that the elements that
help us eat and sleep better can also make us

healthier and happier. This is also the case for the people that we live with, our loved ones. Family members who are involved in the process of creating their own comfort zone tend to achieve more, and this multiplies the effect, making everything extraordinary.

This is a department where DIY effort reaps the maximum outcome, what I call HIME, Highest Impact, Minimum Effort. The process of carrying out any changes and enhancements yourself is also part of the impact that you are putting into the ultimate outcome.

By the end of this chapter, you will understand that there is actual scientific evidence for the common phrase, "beauty sleep." You will also learn how the kitchen and the dining areas in your home form the hearth where relationships are put on the stove to tenderize, so to speak.

STARTING WITH "WHY?"

One fact is so important that it is repeated here although already mentioned before: more than one-third of our lives are spent sleeping.[42]

If we have been created to sleep for one-third of our lives, sleep must be one of the fundamental needs of our being. So, why not fulfil this fundamental need in the most impactful way? The bedroom is for sleeping, sex, and a bit of reading. I always add, jokingly, "not for Netflix, Amazon, or online grocery shopping." Having awareness of the true purpose of the bedroom is a critical detail of our everyday well-being. As much as we might not be able to commit to fully abstaining from technology in the bedroom, it is wise to be aware of it and to have a system of managing the way that we deploy technology in this space.[43]

As for the kitchen and the dining area, do you remember the times when you hosted friends or spent time with your own family over dinner, sitting down where you are most comfortable, either in the living room or making a meal in the kitchen, or over the dining table?

The overarching learning that is important is the differentiation of the technical activity versus the effectual and ultimate reason why we carry out the activity. To sleep is to restore, to cook or dine is to bond.

THE SPIRE DEFINITION OF
WHOLE WELL-BEING

According to do to Dr Tal Ben-Shahar's SPIRE model of happiness, which he teaches at the Happiness Studies Academy,[44] happiness can be understood to be a composite of five aspects of well-being, forming what he calls whole well-being:

S is for spiritual well-being;

P is for physical well-being;

I is for intellectual well-being;

R is for relational well-being; and

E is for emotional well-being.

Each of these facets of well-being and happiness can be paid attention to through our daily activities and the way that we live our lives.

Spiritual well-being is not necessarily about religion, but is more about the way that we manage our state of mind, the way that we are able to see well-being as a result of the ways that our brain functions and controls our emotions and responses. For me, being spiritually well is about anchoring my every living moment to be a servant. Through my commitment to serving a bigger goal of delivering good, my mental state is calibrated at a level that helps me experience serenity and be without unnecessary pressure and anxiety.

Physical well-being is easier to understand, but what is often overlooked in physical well-being is the need for restorative care.

Intellectual well-being is related to growth and learning. The constant quest for skills and knowledge forms one of the key pillars of how a state of happiness can be gradually attained and advanced. This principle is very closely related to the concept of Growth+Learning (G of EGM) explained in the preceding chapter.

I am a firm believer of Marian Diamond's "use it or lose it" principle, and will never shy away from learning new things. Hence my active pursuit of learning and sharing music. To me, this is partly indulgence and partly a way to expand my repertoire of service to share even more broadly.

Relational well-being is linked to the way that we built relationships, and being in those relationship helps us to be present and promotes our happiness.

My constant work-in-progress to battle against depression is underpinned by the urge and motivation to sustain and build a stronger bond with my daughters. It is of key importance to me to have the best relationship I can have with them every day. My relationship with my daughters is what gives my life Meaning+Purpose (that is, the M of EGM).

Emotional well-being is linked to the science of understanding the ways that our brain functions, particularly the way the brain creates hormones.

When I started to write this book, I stopped relying on the medications I had depended on daily for two and a half years. I have since built new habits and routines that work for me, and I am proud to say that I am emotionally balanced. Not only do I not have roller coaster emotional rides, but I am constantly in a balanced and healthy state.

The Happiness Study Academy's principles of SPIRE can be cross-linked to three spaces that I would like to describe.

These spaces are DKZzzz:

1. The dining table;
2. The kitchen; and
3. The bedroom.

KITCHEN AND DINING CREATE DIFFERENT FEELINGS

The kitchen is a place where we do a lot of things. It is not a food preparation machine space, it is not a factory line that creates nutrition, but it is where we often spend time together to prepare nourishment for our physical bodies. The kitchen is where we can focus on and build on our relational well-being and our physical well-being, alongside the activity of preparing food.

Making food together is a significant way to enhance relational well-being. As well as building bonds by sharing common experiences, scientific experiments have shown that food that has been prepared with love tastes better.[45] Food, of course, also nourishes the physical body, promoting our physical well-being.

The dining table is not simply a space where your plates, cups and glasses rest, together with your cutlery. You do not simply consume food at the dining table. In my mind, the dining space is where the most stimulating and heart-warming conversations and bonding occurs. Here we form and deepen relationships, teaching each other a deeper understanding and an appreciation of the relevance of emotional well-being. This is done through conversations and the sharing of insights and deepest thoughts.

Over my dining table, I have enjoyed the deepest and most philosophical conversations with my two young daughters. Perhaps those insights might not qualify to become papers that can be published in philosophical journals, but I gained insights and had many opportunities to connect with my daughters at a deep level.

BEDROOM
YOUR COMFORT ZONE

One of the most intimate and personal spaces in your home is your bedroom, and here, in your sanctuary for your most private and quietest moments, is also where you can attain spiritual well-being. We often overlook the bedroom and see it as a multi-functioning space where we also work, as many people did during (and have done so since) the COVID-19 pandemic. It is, however, a place that has to be prepared with deep care and an acute sensibility. Given the chance, the bedroom is where you can calm your mind, quietening your mental state to attain the alpha and the beta brain states of meditation. It is where you can find solace and process your day. In the bedroom, the easiest hack to make the bedroom function better is to reduce the wifi signal. The best-case scenario, of course, is to agree to leave our devices outside the bedroom, but we know that often this is not possible.

A sizeable chunk of my intake of knowledge through reading is done in my bedroom. Where do you do yours? Reading, preferably from a physical book, also has the effect of moving our brains into a frequency that is more like our original (think cavemen) mode of mental calm.

The benefits of the pre-sleep routine[46] is one of the most significant research findings of recent years, and it is important that we invest time to make sure that the activity that we do for one-third of our entire lives fulfils its core mission and purpose.

THE SPACE YOU CREATE FOR REST AND FAMILY TIME IS AS IMPORTANT FOR WELL-BEING

The way that your dining table is designed is important. I have two of them, one that we use every day, and another that has an extension that can be utilised for larger gatherings.

I have designed my dining table using birch ply for the tabletop, and have used this material specifically because it has the property of being rather soft and easy to mark.

This kind of surface speaks to my feel-good factor. I am drawn to this surface, and I don't feel bad if there are marks on it, as these marks signify moments that have brought me great joy. They add to my sense of well-being, acting as triggers to help me remember times spent with loved ones.

It wasn't my idea to leave marks on the table: in fact, it came from my daughter. When my family and I were thinking about how we would like the dining table to look, the design was decided in consultation with my youngest daughter. She gave me an interesting insight into how we ought to look at the surfaces we eat on. We decided that we would leave the tabletop untreated, exposing it to being marked and showing spills. These red wine and food spills are markers, like the way that we have stamps in our passports of the countries we visit. They record moments of meals that were had around this table and, according to my daughter, this is the best way to build memories.

FEED NOT THE STOMACH
BUT THE SOUL

Our kitchen is also an area of well-being. In Asia, we often have to enclose our kitchens because of the type of cooking methods we use. But we also know that this is another space where the most interesting and intimate conversations are had. While cooking we talk about many things beyond cooking. Family involvement, in terms of conversations along with the actual task of cooking, is the second function of any kitchen. For me, my fondest memories surrounding food and meals are those occasions when I was making the meal together with whoever I am with. The extension of the time interacting and co-creating plates of food we put on the table is far more experientially sumptuous then just the meal alone.

CURATE YOUR SPACE

For the dining area and the kitchen to positively impact the various elements which make up your personal and your family's well-being, you should proactively curate and make these spaces work for you. Look at how dinners are made and eaten. When possible, look into scheduling meals that can be prepared together. This might be as elaborate as having a bake-off day, or as simple as the joint preparation of sandwiches.

One of the details that we have to bear in mind in today's environment is to eliminate or at least reduce the way that our attention is frequently and intermittently drawn to our devices.

BOTTOM LINE

We shape the spaces in our own homes, and they, in turn, shape us. These spaces are the locations of our daily habits and our daily habits influence the way that we function. The spaces are like vessels for the activities that happen within them, and it is not so much the technical movements, but rather the enhancing of the relationships that can be attained through the activities. By careful observation, you can curate your space to improve your well-being and happiness.

TRY THIS OUT

Start with a minimum of one family dinner together each week. During the family dinner, spend between 20 minutes and an hour together without technology or TV. Increase the weekly number of family dinners to a number agreed by the whole family. This requires the entire family to be committed to the agreed number of dinners together. I would recommend you have two or three weekly dinners as a minimum.

In the bedroom, it is important to address your pre-sleep routines, including couples actually scheduling intimate time together. For sleep quality, I recommend the control of your light source and if necessary, the use of additional controlling devices such as lighting that has been designed with circadian considerations, as well as installing motorized roller blinds. When detailed and installed well, these blinds can provide a room that is free from light, allowing you to better align with your natural circadian rhythm. Combined with this, a good-quality circadian rhythm bedside reading light would allow you to enjoy a favourite book and let the mind settle into a gentle pre-sleep routine.

UP NEXT ...

The next thing we are going to talk about is the urgent need to propagate the WHAD movement in today's society. I believe that by making simple hacks and making them everyday habits which you speak about, we are upgrading humanity in a small but big way. There is compelling evidence that deliberate planning towards actions increases our well-being exponentially.

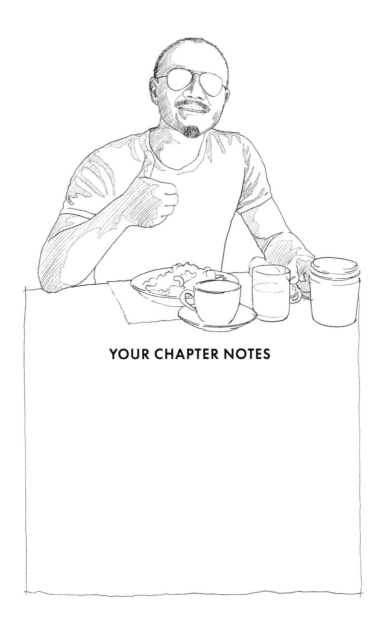

YOUR CHAPTER NOTES

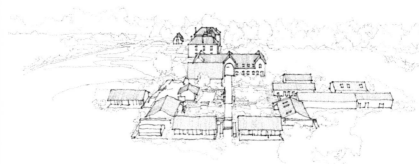

DRAWING: THE OVERALL AERIAL VIEW OF BONNEVAUX MEDITATION CENTRE
(IN POITIER, FRANCE), INCLUDING ITS LATER EXPANSION PHASES.

CHAPTER 10

HOW TO WHAD AHEAD?

"A SMALL GROUP OF THOUGHTFUL PEOPLE COULD CHANGE THE WORLD."

MARGARET MEAD

If I believe that WHAD is a field that can boost any individual's well-being, it would be selfish of me to share it only with a select few. Like many good things in the universe, sharing well-being and happiness through architecture and design (WHAD) is not a zero-sum game. The urge is to propagate it in all shapes and forms, distributing this magic dust even to strangers we might meet on the train.

I am a keen advocate for life to be lived abundantly. The mantra that I repeat to myself, and that I suggest and encourage others to abide by, is: Don't just survive, live your life. It puzzles me that many people I talk to tell me that they have no deep-rooted purpose and feel life is a journey to endure, and they have barely enough energy to survive. Having no clear target, no mission or purpose, will not help steer each of us towards living every day meaningfully.

"DON'T JUST SURVIVE, LIVE YOUR LIFE."

I came to realise how we live daily is a crucial investment in our mental and physical well-being. That's when I came up with the WHAD Movement and the belief that the WHAD concept is not very different to a simple good code of living every day in full presence. The only difference is that the concept of WHAD has more focus and therefore a greater potential to empower oneself towards action. We can form good habits which in turn contribute to us leading good lives. These habits become, over time, a state of sustained elevated well-being within our surroundings.

Your elevated well-being will positively impact those around you. You will discover that aligning your personal space with well-being concepts and principles will lead to more positive energy with the people you come across, especially your dearest ones, in your living and work environments.

We focus on simple changes and tasks that are absolutely within your control. On a spiritual well-being front, this process also educates us to be aware of how our environment makes us feel, and how it can operate more effectively every day.

Have you ever felt like everything that you have experienced and gone through up to this very moment in time was a plan for something bigger? A larger cause? A more ambitious goal? My experiences over the last 10 to 15 years have led me to understand how important it is to channel my own energy towards a goal and a purpose much bigger than myself.

This is not a book about me proclaiming that I have the power to change the world, although I am announcing that I am interested to make every effort and to invest every ounce of energy I have towards that. I have grown my technical and base architectural and design expertise over the last 25 years, and I now commit and dedicate the second half of my life to promoting an unusual and special ethos.

The WHAD Movement is our effort to connect well-being to our fundamental human instinct for happiness. I am addressing this through the lens of architecture and design. We spend 90% of our daily lives inside buildings. The remaining 10% is mostly in other forms of man-made environments, outside buildings but nonetheless constructed. The way spaces mean to us and relate to us, both consciously and subconsciously, is both abundantly magical and powerful.

A well-designed environment can make us feel calm, and a harmoniously curated sequence of rooms and spaces can give us sensorial pleasure or provide education and experiences. The delicately considered balance of nature's signatures in a built environment brings a heightened awareness of our existence as human beings on planet Earth.

Coupled with technology, all this knowledge and possible manifestations are endless. It is not limited by geography or culture. After all, well-being and happiness are abundant and for all of us to tap into.

This book shows us the mental framework to enable us to appreciate how our senses, our preferences, and our personal inclinations are the key ingredients that give us the current relational understanding of the spaces we dwell in.

PURPOSEFUL LIVING

Our homes can be designed to suit our comfort level and enhance our creativity. If we are in a state of well-being, we will be able to come up with solutions and ideas to face daily challenges and lead enriched lives. Lately, my goal for WHAD is to widen its visibility and explain its importance. Getting out of bed every morning with a mission motivates me to be positive. This is how I feel we should lead our everyday lives: purposefully and positively.

Do you have a personal statement of what you stand for? For me, it is to make a difference in the world using the skills and blessings I have been granted thus far. Using my insights and experience in design and architecture, both in the realm of conceptual thinking as well as in team and practice management, I want to put all my accumulated experience and knowledge toward something purposeful.

Putting this to use in thinking about how I can attain well-being and happiness is a sheer delight. When I moved into my new home after the pandemic lockdowns, I channelled all the energy I had in reserve towards the makeover of my new place. This daily activity of thinking about and being hands-on, creating what I came up with, became the reason I got out of bed every day with enthusiasm.

As time passes, our everyday habits and patterns adapt and change. When we observe these signs, we should consider making changes to the space(s) surrounding us. A friend shared that her son, who had slept in the same bedroom from childhood until he graduated from university, felt stuck. By the time he was in his twenties, whenever he entered that room, he felt that he was back in time and that he couldn't move forward. He had childhood memories locked in the colour, design, and small details of the room. Eventually, he moved out and rented his own place. He is now successful in his chosen career. He designed his own space the way he wanted it to be: minimalistic, with wood and white walls. This space helped him be an independent balanced adult, with better family relationships. We need to curate our space based on our state of being at different ages of our lives.

Slowly but surely, I have completed much of the work in my own home with my own two hands, and the satisfaction of seeing this process through, from images in my mind to physical spaces that allow me to enjoy time with my loved ones, fill me with a sense of accomplishment. I feel the future is full of joy and hope.

In a recent LinkedIn post I shared a clip made some 12 months ago of my manifesto. I'm proud that nothing has changed. I'm comfortable within myself, albeit now I look slightly different with my head shaved. If any-thing, the "how" of my achieving this auda-cious ambition to make a dent in the universe is now so much clearer.

GET MOVING

For the WHAD movement to have influence, it is important that you become increasingly sensitive and observant about all the personal spaces that you interact with, and empower yourself with the ability to make informed changes, whether large or small. If these changes lead to better sleep, to having bet-ter family support, if you experience stronger emotional connections with everyone near you, this is due, at least in part, to the spaces in which these events happened.

You are encouraged to launch your life of purpose through the lens of the WHAD movement. Perhaps I should paraphrase that: It is a necessary obligation to yourself and those near you that you understand the prin-ciples of WHAD, and to promote the features of WHAD that you have learned through this book to every single person around you.

I invite you to join the movement using the link and the QR code provided herein. I welcome you to the tribe, and I am pleased that the app platform is another format where we can share what we have learned on a daily basis. I call this the A to Zs of WHAD. My call to action to you is to journal once a week from now on, writing down one thing that you have done for yourself as part of the WHAD movement.

Alongside the launch of this book, I am committed to intensify my contribution to humanity, through all channels and mediums that are within my reach. These will include talks, workshops, and more articles online. I hope to see everyone, you and those you influence today, in any, if not all of these forums. Until then, enjoy your amazing quest for well-being and happiness.

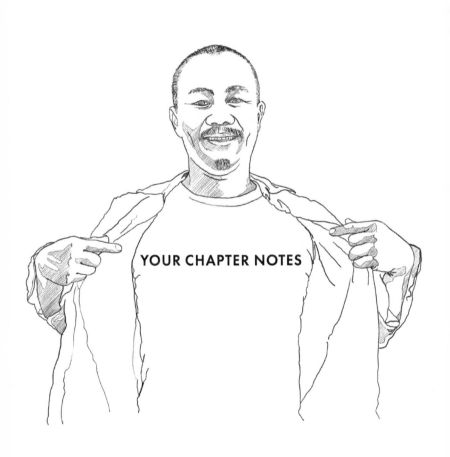

"YOUR TIME IS LIMITED, SO DON'T WASTE IT LIVING SOMEONE ELSE'S LIFE. DON'T BE TRAPPED BY DOGMA – WHICH IS LIVING WITH THE RESULTS OF OTHER PEOPLE'S THINKING."

STEVE JOBS

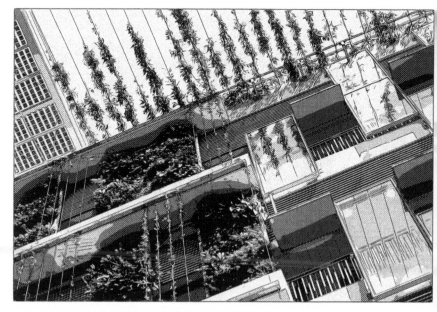

PHOTO: LOOK-UP VIEW OF DETAILS AT THE ATRIUM OF CLEANTECH ONE, SINGAPORE.

Source: Author's own collection

CONCLUSION

I would like to continue to do my work to inspire both myself and everyone that I reach to believe that we can actually make a dent in the universe. We need only take baby steps, so long as they are in the right direction, to progress towards making this dent. Small, but ultimately big steps.

In all our various modes of existing and functioning within humanity, we all dwell in this outer shell of built form and environment. When this built environment is conceived and created sensitively, with an informed mind to enhance well-being, we have a much better chance of growing our relationships in a positive way.

I am excited that many of the insights that I have been gathering for a period of more than five years are now collected in this book. Writing this book has helped me and I truly believe that reading it will be of assistance to you, the reader. I am thrilled that I am on the journey of my Small but Big (aka #SBB) WHAD Movement.

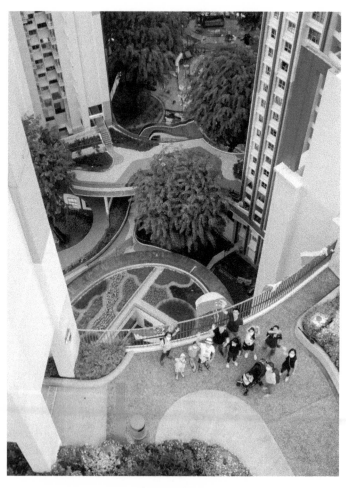

PHOTO: 2022 MEETUP OF (MOST OF) THE ORIGINAL DESIGN TEAM
WHO HELPED MY CONCEPTUALIZED THE MEGA HOUSING PROJECT OF
SKY RESIDENCES (AKA NEW GENERATION HOUSING), SINGAPORE.

FOR THE ARCHITECTURE
AND DESIGN FRATERNITY

COVID-19 TAUGHT US THAT
HEALTH IS WEALTH

Being a designer delivering positive impacts
to everyday living is a great blessing. When
one is granted such an opportunity, there is
also the need for commitment to do it well.

*"WITH GREAT POWER COMES
GREAT RESPONSIBILITY."[47]*

SPIDERMAN

In the fast-paced and competitive realm of
architecture, firms must continually adapt
to stay ahead. Two primary strategies have
emerged in response to this challenge: competing on fees by charging less, and emphasis-
ing the quality of work, often enabling higher
fees. Although both approaches have merits,
the key is to strike a balance that preserves
the essence of architectural services: creating
environments that bring joy, calm, and well-
being to their occupants. This has become
particularly relevant since the COVID-19
pandemic, which underscored the meaning
of the adage, "Health is wealth."

Competing on fees offers a seemingly attractive proposition, especially for firms seeking a foothold in the market, or aiming to secure new clients rapidly. By lowering prices, architects may entice a larger clientele and expand their portfolio, generating more revenue. However, this approach carries significant risks. Charging less may necessitate compromising the time and attention devoted to each project, resulting in lower commitment and ultimately affecting the work's overall quality.

Conversely, concentrating on elevating the quality of work allows architects to showcase their expertise, creativity, and meticulous attention to detail. This approach often leads to innovative, tailored solutions addressing each client's unique needs, enabling firms to charge higher fees and fostering a reputation for excellence. However, challenges accompany this approach as well. Prioritizing high-quality work necessitates significant investments in time, resources, and personnel. Moreover, architects may face mounting pressure to innovate and differentiate themselves in an ever-evolving market. In my experience, focus on quality can be built upon the teaching of the client's own awareness and understanding, which this book is intended to do.

DESIGN ENTERPRISE

To flourish in the competitive architectural landscape, firms must balance these two strategies. I call this the Design Enterprise approach: Design first and allow the business half to flow naturally. To me, excellence in design and execution should remain a priority.

It is crucial to remember that an architect or designer's fundamental mission is to create spaces that are centered on the needs of the users and occupants. The pandemic has highlighted the importance of prioritizing health and well-being in built environments. Therefore, architects must integrate these considerations into their work, emphasizing the creation of human-centric designs that cater to their occupants' physical and emotional needs.

MAKE OUR MEANS TO MAKE A LIVING EVEN MORE DIFFICULT?

Teaching laypersons the acumen and sensibilities to understand and decipher design details can be the best education we give the world.

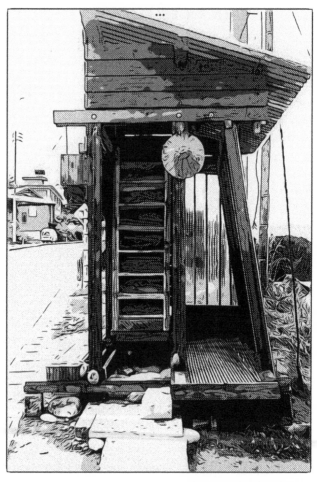

PHOTO: BUS-STOP IN THE REMOTE KOSHIRAURA VILLAGE IN NIIGATA
PREFECTURE OF JAPAN. DESIGN AND BUILT DURING A 3-WEEK SUMMER
WORKSHOP IN 1997 WITH TUTOR SHIN EGASHIRA.

Achieving success in the architecture industry requires delivering value-added services that blend creativity, functionality, and well-being. By supporting the WHAD movement, we are nourishing the baseline of the world's knowledge about well-being and happiness. This, in turn, creates the opportunity for architects and designers to punch higher, and aim for greater heights. Such a philosophy is a great deal more constructive and productive, enabling us to produce higher-quality work and nurture more robust long-term client relationships.

Through the WHAD approach, I believe that designers can optimise their skills in integrating health and well-being considerations. Architects can ensure their work remains a testament to the vital role they play in shaping spaces that promote human flourishing. This is a second layer of how we achieve well-being and happiness through architecture and design.

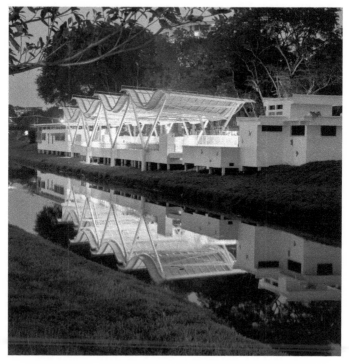

PHOTO: AQUATIC SCIENCE CENTRE, AN ON-SITE RESEARCH FACILITY TO
STUDY URBAN WATERS. LOCATED AT ULU PANDAN, SINGAPORE.

Source: Author's own collectio

FURTHER SUGGESTED READING

(RELEVANT FOR EACH CHAPTER)

Chapter 1 – #SBB: Small but Big

Good Work, by Laurence Freeman, Meditatio (2019).

The Code of the Extraordinary Mind, by Vishen Lakhiani, Rodal Books, Penguin Random House (2019).

The 7 Habits of Highly Effective People, by Stephen Covey, Simon and Schuster (1989).

The Subtle Art of Not Giving a F*ck (A counter Intuitive Way of Living a Good Life), by Mark Manson, Harper Collins Books (2016).

How to find Calm, by Sophie Golding, Sumerside Publishers (2019).

Chapter 2 – The Eureka of WHAD (aka Well-Being+Happiness thru' Architecture+Design)

Start with Why, by Simon Sinek, Penguin Business (2009).

Find your Why, by Simon Sinek with David Mead and Peter Docker, Penguin Business (2017).

The How of Happiness (A Practical Guide to Getting the Life you want), by Sonia Lyubormirsky, Sphere (2007).

The Happiness Advantage. By Shawn Achor, Virgin Books (2010).

Big Potential (Five Secrets of Reaching Higher by Powering those around you), by Shawn Achor, Virgin Books (2018).

Freedom to be Happy (The Business Case for Happiness), by Matthew Phelon, Happiness and Humans Publishing (2020).

The Book of Joy (Lasting Happiness in a Changing World) by His Holiness the Dalai Lama and Archbishop Desmond Tutu, with Douglas Abrams, Hutchinson London, Penguin Random House (2016).

Building Happiness (Architecture to Make You Smile), Edited by Jane Wernick, Black Dog Publishing (2008).

Chapter 3 – Curiosity and Competence

Play (How it shapes the brain, Opens the Imagination and Invigorates the Soul), by Stuart Brown MD, Penguin Group (2010).

The Spiritual Child (The New Science of Parenting for Health and Lifelong Thriving), by Lisa Miller PhD, Bluebird Books for Life (2015).

Counter Clockwise (Mindful Health and the Power of Possibility), by Ellen J. Langer, Ballantine Books (2009).

A Million Things to Ask a Neuroscientist (The brain Made Easy), by Mike Tranter PhD, The English Scientist (2021).

Chapter 4 – Six Senses

Design a Healthy Home (100 ways to transform your space for physical and mental well-being), by Oliver Heath, Dorling Kindersley Ltd, Penguin Random House (2021).

Good Anxiety, by Dr Wendy Suzuki with Billie Fitzpatrick, Atria Books (2021).

Chapter 5 – The Power of Materiality

Happiness by Design (Finding pleasure and Purpose in everyday life), by Paul Dolan, Penguin (2013).

Biomimicry in Architecture, by Michael Pawlyn, RIBA Publishing (2016).

Chapter 6 – Understanding the Functions of Spaces

Neuroscience for Designing Green Spaces, by Agnieszka Olszewska-Guizzo, Routledge (2023).

Happy by Design, by Victoria Harrison, Octopus Publishing Group (2018).

The Happy Design Toolkit (Architecture for Better Mental Wellbeing), by Ben Channon, RIBA Publishing (2022).

The Design of Everyday Things, by Don Norman, Basic Books (2013).

Chapter 7 – Modern Day Cavemen

The Incredible Human Journey (The Story of How We Colonised the Planet), by Alice Roberts, Bloomsbury (2009).

Tamed, by Prof Alice Roberts, Windmill Books, Penguin Random House (2017).

Sapiens (A brief History of Humankind). by Yuval Noah Harari, Vintage, Penguin Random House (2011).

Hardwired for Happiness (9 Proven Practices to Overcome Stress and Live Your Best Life), by Ashish Kothari, Houndstooth Press (2022).

Chapter 8 – Tribes

A Hunter-Gatherer's Guide to the 21st Century, by Heather Heying and Bret Weinstein, Swift (2022).

Homo Deus (A brief History of Tomorrow), by Yuval Noah Harari, Vintage, Penguin Random House (2015).

21 Lessons for the 21st Century by Yuval Noah Harari, Vintage, Penguin Random House (2018).

Chapter 9 – DKZzzz
(Dining/Kitchen/Sleep)

Happiness Studies. By Tal Ben-shahar, Palgrave Macmillan (2021).

Why we sleep, by Mathew Walker, Penguin Books UK (2018).

The Shaping of Us, by Lily Bernheimer, Robinson UK (2017).

Happy Inside, by Michelle Ogundehin, Ebury Press, Penguin Random House (2020).

My Hygge Home (How to make home your Happy Place), by Meik Wiking (2022).

The Great Indoors (The Surprising Science of How Buildings Shape our Behavior, Health and Happiness), by Emily Anthes Scientific American Picador (2021).

The Miracle Morning (The 6 Habits that will Transform Your Life before 8AM), by Hal Elrod, John Murray Learning (2016).

Chapter 10 – How to WHAD Ahead

Architecture for Well Being, by Raman Vig, Adhyyan Books (2021).

Designing for Wellbeing (An Applied Approach), Edited by Ann Petermans and Rebecca Cain, Routledge (2020).

Programming for Health and Wellbeing in Architecture, Edited by Keely Menezes MPH, Pamela de Oliveira-Smith and A. Vernon Woodworth FAIA, Routledge (2022).

The Architecture of Happiness, by Alain De Botton, Penguin (2014).

Mental Health at Work, by James Routledge, Penguin Business (2021).

ADDITIONAL READING ...

Mind in Architecture (Neuroscience, Embodiment and the Future of Design), edited by Sarah Robinson and Juhani Pallasmaa, MIT Press (2017).

NeuroArchitecture, by Christoph Mewtzger, Jovis Books (2018).

The Architect's Brain (Neuroscience, Creativity and Architecture) by Harry Francis Mallgrave, Wiley-Blackwell (2011).

The Little Book of Humanism, by Andrew Copson and Alice Roberts, Platkus, 2020.

Happy Ever After, by Paul Dolan, Penguin (2018).

The Courage to be Happy, by Ichiro Kishimi and Fumitake Koga, Allen & Unwin (2020).

Tiny Habits, by B. J. Fogg PhD, Penguin (2019).

INTERESTING RESEARCH PAPERS

Transitional areas affect perception of workspaces and employee well-being: A study of underground and above-ground workspaces. *Building and Environment, 179*, 106840.

By Tan, Z., Roberts, A. C., Lee, E. H., Kwok, K. W., Car, J., Soh, C. K., & Christopoulos, G. (2020).

Prevalence and factors associated with stress in the workplace in SG: Prevalence of psychological distress and its association with perceived indoor environmental quality and workplace factors in under and aboveground workplaces.

By Dunleavy, G., Bajpai, R., Tonon, A. C., Cheung, K. L., Thach, T. Q., Rykov, Y., ... & Christopoulos, G. (2020). *Building and environment, 175*, 106799.

Experimental study on workplace cubicles: The cubicle deconstructed: Simple visual enclosure improves perseverance.

Roberts, A. C., Yap, H. S., Kwok, K. W., Car, J., Soh, C. K., & Christopoulos, G. I. (2019). *Journal of Environmental Psychology, 63*, 60-73.

Short- and long-term effects of architecture on the brain: Toward theoretical formalization.

Paiva, A., Jedon, R. (2019). *Frontiers of Architectural Research,* 8(4), 564-571. DOI: 10.1016/j. foar.2019.07.004.

How Building Design Can Influence Behaviors and Performance.

Paiva, A. (2018) Neuroscience for Architecture: *Journal of Civil Engineering and Architecture,* 12(2), 132-138. DOI: 10.17265/1934-7359/2018.02.007.

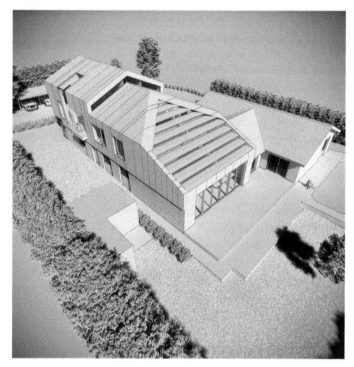

IMAGES: PROPOSAL FOR PRIVATE HOME IN OUTER LONDON, WITH A KEY
DESIGN FEATURE BEING THE CELEBRATION OF NATURAL LIGHT.

Source: Author's own collection

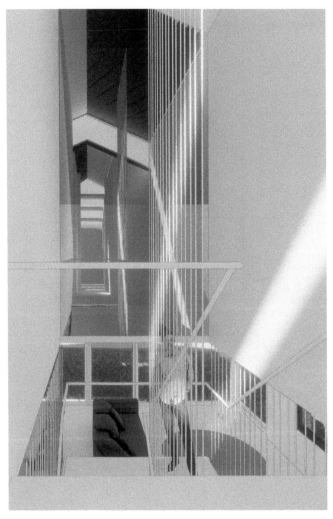

IMAGES: PROPOSAL FOR PRIVATE HOME IN OUTER LONDON, WITH A KEY
DESIGN FEATURE BEING THE CELEBRATION OF NATURAL LIGHT.

Source: Author's own collection

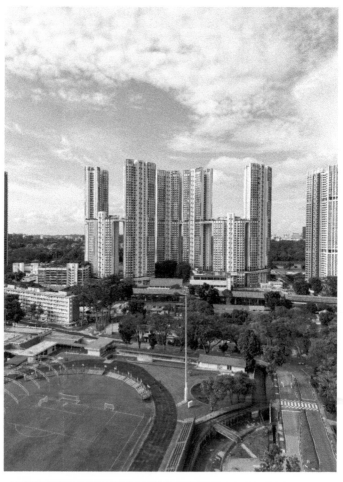

PHOTO: SKY RESIDENCES (AKA NEW GENERATION HOUSING), SINGAPORE.

Source: Author's own collection

AUTHOR BIO

Frven Lim is an expert in the field of holistic well-being design. He combines 25 years of professional architectural knowledge, research findings from various disciplines, and personal insights, to pioneer this emerging specialisation.

His methodology is evident-based and the techniques he uses involve applied research of his own studies as well as adaptations of research by neuroscientists and other human behaviour specialists.

After the COVID-19 pandemic in 2020, he coined #WHAD, which stands for "Well-being+Happiness through Architecture+Design." This movement has since been steadily growing among the tribe of far-sighted architects and designers who believe in the importance of meaning and purpose, as well as the wider mission of an architectural designer's calling.

He champions the motto of "making a difference through design." This is evident in his thought leadership articles and openly accessible webinars on social media platforms. His unique skills lie in the global and human-centric approach to well-being applied research.

As a keen advocate of using creativity as a channel to instigate positive change, he is often invited to speak at webinars and conferences on the topic of how architecture and design affect the inhabitants' well-being and happiness.

There is growing interest and recognition in the real estate industry that WHAD has the power to deliver life and habit-changing products/services that are commercially value-adding in a highly competitive market.

Fundamentally, Frven's mission is to make evident the conduit for designers to fulfil the holistic mission of creating truly better places and spaces. In short, he openly declares that his purpose in life is to elevate humanity's well-being.

TECHNICAL ACHIEVEMENTS

Frven has a built track record in excess of 11,000 residential units and 2 million square meters over the more than two decades of his professional career.

Under a full scholarship from the Singapore government, he trained at the University of Manchester, and next at the Architectural Association in London, where he received his AA diploma in 1999. His outstanding grades led to him being granted a full AA scholarship for him to achieve his MA (Distinction) in the field of Landscape Urbanism in 2001.

He practices with an attitude of experimentation and research. This originality is evident in his works and has earned him several high-profile design awards, including the prestigious "20 under 45" accolade accorded by Singapore's Urban and Redevelopment Authority in 2010.

Throughout his career, Frven has spearheaded design studios in Singapore and London. His repertoire includes projects ranging from the smallest bespoke urban insertions to large-scale townships and masterplans. His diverse portfolio across Asia, the Middle East, India, China, the UK and Europe ranges from private residential, commercial and retail schemes to government/ public commissions.

ACADEMIA AND PUBLICATIONS

In the deepest part of his heart, Frven is a teacher. He has served in many capacities in the architectural design sector, including as an invited tutor/critic for Harvard GSD, Switzerland EPFL and the Architectural School of Singapore NUS.

He has authored and edited numerous publications, including four seminal books are "Housing People," "1degNorth," "Crafting Public Realms" and "Project 2050." In addition, Frven has contributed an essay that was published alongside the exhibition titled "1000+ Singapores" held at Paris' city hall in the summer of 2015.

Publication References:

"20under45: The Next Generation," 2010 (ISBN: 978-981-08-3860-7)

"project 2050," 2014 (ISBN: 978-981-09-2224-5)

"Crafting Public Realms," 2014 (ISBN: 978-981-09-0225-4)

"1degNorth," 2013 (ISBN: 978-981-07-7534-6)

"Housing People," 2012 (ISBN: 978-981-07-1793-3)

FURTHER INFORMATION

Prominent Awards

"20under45: The Next Generation" (2010), selected as one of twenty prominent Singapore registered Architects under the age of 45

Recipient of AA School Masters programme Scholarship, 1999

Recipient of HDB Overseas Scholarship, 1993

Qualifications

WELL Accredited Professional (2021), Int'l Well-being Institute (License No: WELL-AP-0000058732)

Fitwel Ambassador (2021-)

Master of Arts (Distinction) (Landscape Urbanism)

Architectural Association, United Kingdom, 2002

Diploma of the Architectural Association

Architectural Association, United Kingdom, 1999

Bachelor of Arts (Honours)

University of Manchester, United Kingdom, 1996

Professional Associations

Member, Academy of Neuroscience for Architecture (ANFA)

Registered APEC Architect, Singapore, 2015-

Registered Architect, #1914, Board of Architects, Singapore, 2005-

Royal Institute of British Architects, Chartered Member, 2008-

EXTRAS

CONNECT WITH ME AND JOIN THE WHAD TRIBE

By taking the step to become part of the WHAD tribe, you reap the most benefits. You will give yourself the opportunity to become even more enlightened, and more importantly, exchange ideas to up-level both yourselves as well as others. That is the WHAD spirit anyway.

I invite you to join me, so we can support each other on this fantastic journey.

THE WHAD APP

Within the website, you will see the option of downloading and becoming a subscriber to our app.

Here you can find online courses and infuse in deeper insights via my video recordings and also my generously dished out "Happywork."

MY CALENDLY

Calendly.com/frvenlim

This is where you can arrange for live conversations of various kinds with me. I would love to speak with you, and share with you insights about how well-being can be elevated, how your journey of getting happier can be achieved.

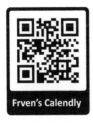

Frven's Calendly

MENTIONED PROJECT/ BUILDING CREDITS

Projects used as illustrations in this book

CleanTech One
(Owner: JTC, Singapore | Architect: Surbana)

Aquatic Science Centre
(Owner: NUS/SDWA, Singapore | Architect: Surbana)

Dawson Sky Residences (aka New Generation Housing Dawson Site C)
(Owner: HDB, Singapore | Architect: Surbana)

Bonneavaux Meditation Centre
(Owner: World Community of Christian Mediators | Architect: DP Architects)

The Biltmore Hotel
(Owner: M&C UK, London | Architect: DP Architects)

Vhi Carrickmines Health Centre
(Owner: Vhi, Dublin | Design Architect: DPA)

stairWELL

(Location: Mediacorp HQ, Singapore |
Research Projected funded by Good Design
Research grant from DesignSingapore)
(Principal Investigator: DPA with Andrea de
Paiva (NeuroAU) and Assoc Prof Georgious
Christopoulos NTU Business School)

ENDNOTES

1 https://en.wikipedia.org/wiki/Butterfly_effect.

2 Watch the film Sliding Doors. See: https://en.wikipedia.org/wiki/Sliding_Doors.

3 Link to LinkedIn post. https://www.linkedin.com/posts/frvenlim_40-years-ago-i-sold-newspapers-i-was-ashamed-activity-6941807541622325248-oDRH?utm_source=share&utm_medium=member_ios.

4 The 7 Habits of Highly Effective People, by Setpeh R. Covey, Simon & Schuster (1989).

5 A short synopsis of this project and the links to online materials is accessible in the format of a video posted here: https://youtu.be/0GGEsZxdX18.

   As well as these LinkedIn posts:

   1. https://www.linkedin.com/posts/frvenlim_stairwell-inactivity-whad-activity-7066416121582641152-Mw_u?utm_source=share&utm_medium=member_ios.

   2. https://www.linkedin.com/posts/frvenlim_the-art-of-stair-climbing-how-to-start-activity-7068179030633521152-jgp4?utm_source=share&utm_medium=member_ios.

6 Info from World Health Organisation: https://www.who.int/data/gho/indicator-metadata-registry/imr-details/3416.

7 See also "unknown unknowns" famously used by Donald Rumsfeld: https://en.wikipedia.org/wiki/There_are_unknown_unknowns.

   Also of interest: https://www.team-consulting.com/insights/dr-design-research-no-donald-rumsfeld/.

8 See articles about Marian Diamond's research, including "Use it or Lose it," https://www.washingtonpost.com/local/obituaries/marian-diamond-neuroscientist-who-gave-new-meaning-to-use-it-or-lose-it-dies-at-90/2017/07/30/ff10060c-752a-11e7-8f39-

eeb7d3a2d304_story.html, and "My Love Affair with the Brain," https://vimeo.com/20125847.

9   See this research publication for more details: https://www.researchgate.net/publication/51389729_Mind-Set_Matters_Exercise_and_the_Placebo_Effect.

10 See further information and resource available at: https://www.limitlessbook.com/.

11 https://knowablemagazine.org/article/health-disease/2020/what-does-a-synapse-do.

12 See "The code of the extraordinary mind" by Vishen Lakhiani (specifically Chapters 1 & 2, pages 3-44).

13 To know more about International WELL Building Institute, see: https://www.wellcertified.com/about-iwbi/.

14 Diagram abstracted from: https://www.researchgate.net/publication/290001505_Lighting_and_health_of_building_occupants_A_case_of_Indian_information_technology_offices#pf2.

15 https://thrivenfunctionalmedicine.com/melatonin-and-cortisol/.

16 https://www.zrtlab.com/blog/archive/cortisol-and-melatonin-in-the-circadian-rhythm/#:~:text=Rising%20cortisol%20in%20the%20morning,increases%20the%20drive%20to%20sleep.

17 https://www.bbc.co.uk/news/health-21572520 and https://www.washington.edu/news/2013/01/02/while-in-womb-babies-begin-learning-language-from-their-mothers/.

18 https://en.wikipedia.org/wiki/Sound_masking.

19 https://www.fooddive.com/news/air-up-scent-flavor-water/627982/#:~:text=%27Flavored%27%20by%20neuroscience&text=What%20makes%20Air%20Up%20work,it%20is%20perceived%20as%20taste.

20 See https://uk.air-up.com.

21 https://direct.mit.edu/jocn/article-abstract/21/8/1523/4714/Recognizing-Threat-A-Simple-Geometric-Shape?redirectedFrom=fulltext.

22 https://bigthink.com/life/fractal-patterns-children/#:~:text=Fractal%20patterns%20can%20reduce%20stress,physiological%20resonance%20within%20the%20eye.

23 https://www.linkedin.com/posts/frvenlim_whadabrfurn-whad-wellbeing-activity-7043476269602107392-E7LG?utm_source=share&utm_medium=member_ios.

24 See diagram. If this interests you, please look up further into this via this link: https://newscenter.lbl.gov/2012/10/17/elevated-indoor-carbon-dioxide-impairs-decision-making-performance/.

25 https://standard.wellcertified.com/water.

26 https://civicscience.com/forty-seven-percent-of-americans-dont-drink-enough-water-plus-more-h2o-insights/#:~:text=The%20latest%20CivicScience%20polling%20shows,drink%20more%20than%20eight%20glasses.

27 About sleep percentage of our lifetime. https://www.linkedin.com/posts/frvenlim_wellbeingdesign-whad-activity-7057700013849632768-lbUE?utm_source=share&utm_medium=member_ios.

28 https://www.dreams.co.uk/sleep-matters-club/your-life-in-numbers-infographic#:~:text=The%20average%20person%20spends%20about,lives%20spent%20asleep%20in%20bed.

29 https://en.wikipedia.org/wiki/Biophilia_hypothesis.

30 https://www.oxfordreference.com/display/10.1093/oi/authority.20110803095507389;jsessionid=7E651D6E587E2BBF5176EC74A682AAF6#:~:text=Love%20of%20life%20and%20living%20things.

31 https://bonnevauxwccm.org.

32 https://rize.io/blog/how-to-avoid-burnout-working-from-home.

33 See related articles such as: https://www.verywellmind.com/news-working-from-home-indefinitely-may-have-hidden-consequences-5084915.

34 https://www.dreams.co.uk/sleep-matters-club/your-life-in-numbers-infographic.

35   HBR Article "How Hardwired Is Human Behavior?"
https://hbr.org/1998/07/how-hardwired-is-human-behavior.

36   Documentary website: https://www.thesocialdilemma.com/

37   To have a deeper understanding of the E+G+M interpretation of Happiness in my personal journey, I invite you to search using the hashtag #EGM in LinkedIn.

38   https://en.wikipedia.org/wiki/Cast_Away.

39   Tribes: We Need You to Lead Us, by Seth Godin, Piatkus Books (2008).

40   https://onlinelibrary.wiley.com/doi/10.1111/j.1468-2494.2008.00477.x.
https://cognitiveresearchjournal.springeropen.com/articles/10.1186/s41235-021-00311-3.

41   Access to "WHAD's A to Z" is available upon signing up to the community, a link to which is included in the closing pages of this book.

42   https://www.dreams.co.uk/sleep-matters-club/your-life-in-numbers-infographic.

43   See https://www.linkedin.com/posts/frvenlim_wellbeingdesign-whad-activity-7057700013849632768-1bUE?utm_source=share&utm_medium=member_ios.

44   https://www.happinessstudies.academy.

45   https://podcasts.ufhealth.org/a-pinch-of-love-really-does-make-food-taste-better/.

46   https://publications.kon.org/urc/v10/garner.html.

47   https://en.wikipedia.org/wiki/With_great_power_comes_great_responsibility#:~:text=%22With%20great%20power%20comes%20great,to%20the%20young%20Peter%20Parker.

NOTES